Catherine J. Hunter
Editor

Controversies in Pediatric Appendicitis

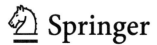 Springer

Editor
Catherine J. Hunter
Feinberg School of Medicine
Northwestern University
Chicago, IL
USA

Ann and Robert H. Lurie Children's Hospital of Chicago
Chicago, IL
USA

ISBN 978-3-030-15005-1   ISBN 978-3-030-15006-8   (eBook)
https://doi.org/10.1007/978-3-030-15006-8

This Springer imprint is published by the registered company Springer Nature Switzerland AG
The registered company address is: Gewerbestrasse 11, 6330 Cham, Switzerland

Preface

Appendicitis is among the most common surgical diseases, and has been a recognized condition for over a century, Despite providing care to a high volume of patients, numerous areas of controversy exist in the management of pediatric appendicitis. Debate exists on every topic from the appropriate nomenclature to the optimal choice of antibiotics. And the decision as to the best surgical approach or whether surgery is even indicated is an area of active research. In this publication, an expert group of physicians and surgeons have come together to provide up-to-date discussions of the key areas of controversy in this field. We believe that this is an excellent addition to the literature providing a crucial reference for all providers and surgeons that care for children with appendicitis.

Chicago, IL, USA   Catherine J. Hunter

Contents

Contributors

Natasha R. Ahuja Department of Surgery, University at Buffalo Jacobs School of Medicine and Biomedical Sciences, Buffalo, NY, USA

John Aiken Children's Hospital of Wisconsin, Milwaukee, WI, USA

Medical College of Wisconsin, Wauwatosa, WI, USA

K. Tinsley Anderson Center for Surgical Trials and Evidence-Based Practice, McGovern Medical School at The University of Texas Health Science Center at Houston, Houston, TX, USA

Guillermo Ares Department of Surgery, University of Illinois at Chicago, Chicago, IL, USA

Leo Andrew Benedict Children's Mercy Hospital, Kansas City, MO, USA

Christie Buonpane Ann & Robert H. Lurie Children's Hospital of Chicago, Chicago, IL, USA

Northwestern University, Chicago, IL, USA

Young Mee Choi Children's Hospital Colorado, Aurora, CO, USA

Rutgers New Jersey Medical School, Newark, NJ, USA

Emily D. Dubina Department of Surgery, Harbor-UCLA Medical Center, Torrance, CA, USA

Dalya M. Ferguson Center for Surgical Trials and Evidence-Based Practice, McGovern Medical School at The University of Texas Health Science Center at Houston, Houston, TX, USA

Christopher Gayer Department of Surgery, Division of Pediatric Surgery, Keck School of Medicine of University of Southern California, Los Angeles, CA, USA

Children's Hospital of Los Angeles, Los Angeles, CA, USA

Seth Goldstein Ann & Robert H. Lurie Children's Hospital of Chicago, Chicago, IL, USA

Northwestern University, Chicago, IL, USA

Robyn M. Hatley Department of Surgery, Medical College of Georgia at Augusta University, Augusta, GA, USA

Section of Pediatric Surgery, Children's Hospital of Georgia, Augusta, GA, USA

Catherine J. Hunter Feinberg School of Medicine, Northwestern University, Chicago, IL, USA

Ann and Robert H. Lurie Children's Hospital of Chicago, Chicago, IL, USA

Marcus Jarboe Departments of Surgery and Vascular and Interventional Radiology, Mott Children's Hospital, University of Michigan, Ann Arbor, MI, USA

Randi L. Lassiter Department of Surgery, Medical College of Georgia at Augusta University, Augusta, GA, USA

Timothy B. Lautz Feinberg School of Medicine, Northwestern University, Chicago, IL, USA

Ann & Robert H. Lurie Children's Hospital of Chicago, Chicago, IL, USA

Steven L. Lee Division of Pediatric Surgery, Mattel Children's Hospital at the University of California, Los Angeles Medical Center, Westwood, CA, USA

Francois I. Luks Division of Pediatric Surgery, Warren Alpert Medical School of Brown University, Hasbro Children's Hospital, Providence, RI, USA

Raoud Marayati Department of Surgery, University of Alabama at Birmingham, Birmingham, AL, USA

Colin Martin Department of Surgery, Division of Pediatric Surgery, University of Alabama at Birmingham, Birmingham, AL, USA

Demetri J. Merianos Department of Surgery, Division of Pediatric Surgery, New York-Presbyterian/Weill Cornell Medical Center, New York, NY, USA

Julie Monteagudo Division of Pediatric Surgery, Warren Alpert Medical School of Brown University, Hasbro Children's Hospital, Providence, RI, USA

Steven Moulton Children's Hospital Colorado, Aurora, CO, USA

University of Colorado School of Medicine, Aurora, CO, USA

Michelle V. L. Nguyen Department of Surgery, Division of Pediatric Surgery, Keck School of Medicine of University of Southern California, Los Angeles, CA, USA

Children's Hospital of Los Angeles, Los Angeles, CA, USA

Alexander W. Peters Department of Surgery, Division of Pediatric Surgery, New York-Presbyterian/Weill Cornell Medical Center, New York, NY, USA

Shawn J. Rangel Department of Pediatric and Thoracic Surgery, Boston Children's Hospital, Boston, MA, USA

Harvard Medical School, Boston, MA, USA

David H. Rothstein Department of Surgery, University at Buffalo Jacobs School of Medicine and Biomedical Sciences, Buffalo, NY, USA

Department of Pediatric Surgery, John R. Oishei Children's Hospital, Buffalo, NY, USA

Sara Smolinski-Zhao Departments of Surgery and Vascular and Interventional Radiology, Mott Children's Hospital, University of Michigan, Ann Arbor, MI, USA

Shawn D. St. Peter Children's Mercy Hospital, Kansas City, MO, USA

Cynthia Susai Division of Pediatric Surgery, Warren Alpert Medical School of Brown University, Hasbro Children's Hospital, Providence, RI, USA

KuoJen Tsao Center for Surgical Trials and Evidence-Based Practice, McGovern Medical School at The University of Texas Health Science Center at Houston, Houston, TX, USA

History and Epidemiology of Pediatric Appendicitis

Guillermo Ares and Catherine J. Hunter

Introduction

Appendicitis is one of the most common surgical conditions treated in children of all ages. While the appendix was identified and grossly described centuries ago, diseases of the appendix were only recognized a little over 100 years ago. Historic terms such as "perityphlitis" were phased out as we began to understand the pathophysiology and histopathologic changes of acute appendicitis. However, as new definitions emerged, so did new questions. The management of appendicitis in children has been hotly debated since the first surgical therapy was described. Currently, novel operative technology, improved antibiotics, and advanced diagnostic instruments have made their way into the treatment algorithms, shedding insight while also inviting along with them more controversies in the management of pediatric appendicitis.

The Dark Ages (Pre-Fitz Era)

The appendix was described as early as 1492 by Leonardo da Vinci, though his drawings were not published until several centuries later. Therefore, the Italian anatomist Berengario da Carpi is credited with the first description of the appendix in 1521 as an "empty small cavity at the end of the cecum" [1]. His words were validated by Andreas Vesalius in his illustrations of the colon published in 1543 in *De*

G. Ares
Department of Surgery, University of Illinois at Chicago, Chicago, IL, USA

C. J. Hunter (✉)
Feinberg School of Medicine, Northwestern University, Chicago, IL, USA

Ann and Robert H. Lurie Children's Hospital of Chicago, Chicago, IL, USA
e-mail: chunter@luriechildrens.org

© Springer Nature Switzerland AG 2019
C. J. Hunter (ed.), *Controversies in Pediatric Appendicitis*,
https://doi.org/10.1007/978-3-030-15006-8_1

Humani Corporis Fabrica. Shortly thereafter, with a graphic representation available and textual description of the appendix, Gabriel Fallopius compared the appendix to a worm, coining the term "the vermiform appendix" [2]. In the ensuing century, sparse reports of inflammation around the area of the appendix appeared, moving the conversations about the appendix from descriptive anatomy to abnormal findings. In 1711, Heister, an alumnus of Boerhaave, described autopsy findings corresponding to a perforated appendix in the right lower quadrant [2]. Several other authors contributed their postmortem findings in the 1700s such as a blackened appendix, a narrow appendix with abscess, and an obstructed appendix with hardened stool in it. Mestivier described an appendix perforated by a pin and surrounded by "a pint of pus" at the right of the umbilicus [3].

In 1812, John Parkinson presented the case of a 5-year-old with a fecalith leading to perforated appendix with a normal cecum, and in 1813, the first description of pediatric acute appendicitis was presented [4]. Wegeler detailed the clinical presentation and hospital course prior to the demise of an 18-year-old patient with 3 days of abdominal pain, diarrhea, and emesis. Wegeler found a gangrenous cecum with an appendix that was "red, enlarged, and filled with stones" [2]. These two cases marked an important transition where the focus started shifting from postmortem analysis to clinical observations in vivo of the diseases of the appendix. Given this and several other reports of fecal peritonitis, Francois Melier suggested the appendix as the source of the problem and appendectomy as a possible treatment [5]. However, his suggestions fell on deaf ears because the influential Guillaume Dupuytren strongly believed that the inflammatory process began in the cecum and not the appendix. Thanks to Dupuytren, the term perityphlitis continued to be the diagnosis given until the late 1880s [6].

During this time period of discovery, the first appendectomy was performed, though acute appendicitis was not the indication for surgery. In 1735, Claudius Amyand performed the first appendectomy in London. His patient was an 11-year-old boy who was admitted for the repair of a congenital inguinal hernia that had progressed to the point of suppurating a discharge of "an unkindly sort of matter" for 1 month [7]. Amyand found an indirect inguinal hernia containing the appendix, which had been perforated by a pin that the boy swallowed. He describes that "many unsuspected oddities" were found, as his assistants held the boy down during this procedure in the preanesthetic era. Challenging as it was, Amyand's patient survived the first surgery of the appendix.

Renaming and Reframing

While the anatomy of the appendix was recognized early, it had no impact on clinical practice until the 1880s. The modern history of acute appendicitis began in 1886 when Reginald Fitz, pathologist at Harvard, read his paper "Perforating Inflammation of the Vermiform Appendix: With Special Reference to Its Early Diagnosis and Treatment" [8]. This landmark article detailed the presentations of 257 cases of appendicitis, emphasizing that the inflammation in the right lower quadrant, commonly misdiagnosed as perityphlitis, in fact originated from the appendix. In the same year, Robert Hall performed the first appendectomy for perforated appendicitis in the United States. Three years later, Charles McBurney entered the fray in 1889 and demanded that the "so-called pericecal inflammation" be referred to as appendicitis, functionally removing the term perityphlitis from the medical jargon [9]. McBurney described in detail the constellation of symptoms that we now associate with "classic" appendicitis. He is perhaps better known for his famous depiction of McBurney's point [9]:

> And I believe that in every case the seat of greatest pain, determined by the pressure of one finger, has been very exactly between an inch and a half and two inches from the anterior spinous process of the ilium on a straight line drawn from that process to the umbilicus.

Surgical removal of the appendix became increasingly popular, as surgeons published overwhelmingly positive results with this procedure. McBurney wrote a very detailed case series of 11 patients including their varying clinical presentation and intraoperative findings. He emphasized that the clinical presentation may not match the severity of the disease, and therefore, he firmly recommended immediate operation for all cases. Others, such as Ochsner in 1902, were not as enthusiastic about operating in perforated appendicitis [10]. Ochsner proposed non-operative treatment for peritonitis, with enemas, gastric lavage, and bowel rest, followed by interval appendectomy. This heated debate continued for the better part of the century and, one could argue, still permeates our discussions today. In 1904, John McMurphy added his opinion by reporting his experience with 2000 appendectomies, publishing the largest case series to date and advocating for immediate appendectomy in support of McBurney's stance, given his low mortality rates [11]. But perhaps the most instrumental event in promoting the surgical treatment of appendicitis was the experience of Sir Frederick Treves. He was summoned by King Edward in 1902 to evaluate him for right lower quadrant pain merely 2 weeks prior to the coronation [12]. The king refused surgical intervention prior to the coronation, which led to a moribund king undergoing abscess drainage weeks later. In the end, he attended the coronation, knowledge of acute appendicitis was publicly disseminated, and appendectomy became the widely accepted treatment.

As a result, the ambition of the era quickly became perfecting surgical technique and mastering the art of surgery. A wide array of surgical approaches were used including transverse laparotomy; midline, paramedian, lateral rectus incisions; oblique incision over the external oblique; and muscle splitting versus cutting incisions [13]. McBurney reported using a right lower quadrant muscle splitting incision. This approach was first used by McArthur, who was unable to present his findings before McBurney. While McBurney admitted this incision was McArthur's, it was his eponymous name that prevailed. Besides the surgical approach, variations on the technique for the removal of the appendix ranged from simple ligation to purse string on the cecum, crushing at the base with serosal oversewing, or imbrication into the cecum, to name a few [14]. With the vanishing of perityphlitis as a diagnosis, surgeons also encouraged physicians to turn away from dated remedies such as cathartics, which only delayed definitive care. Therefore, the history of appendicitis progressed from naming an unnamed disease to improving treatment and minimizing harm.

3. Seal A. Appendicitis: a historical review. Can J Surg. 1981;24(4):427–33.
4. Major RH. Classic descriptions of disease, with biographical sketches of the authors. 3rd ed. Springfield: C. C. Thomas; 1945. p. 651–2.
5. de Moulin D. Historical notes on appendicitis. Arch Chir Neerl. 1975;27(2):97–102.
6. Stewart D. The management of acute appendicitis. In: Cameron JL, Cameron AM, editors. Current surgical therapy. 11th ed. Philadelphia: Elsevier Saunders; 2014.
7. Amyand C. Of an inguinal rupture, with a pin in the appendix caeci, incrusted with stone; and some observations on wounds in the guts. Philos Trans R Soc Lond. 1735;39:329–36.
8. Fitz R. On perforating inflammation of the vermiform appendix with special reference to its early diagnosis and treatment. N Engl J Med. 1935;213(6):245–8.
9. McBurney C. Experience with early operative interference in cases of disease of the vermiform appendix. N Y Med J. 1889;50:676–84.
10. Ochsner AJ. A handbook of appendicitis. Chicago: G.P. Engelhard & Co; 1902. p. 182.
11. Meade RH. The evolution of surgery for appendicitis. Surgery. 1964;55:741–52.
12. Treves F. The Cavendish lecture on some phases of inflammation of the appendix: delivered before the West London Medico-Chirurgical Society on June 20th, 1902. Br Med J. 1902;1(2165):1589–94.
13. Strohl EL, Diffenbaugh WG. The historical background of the gridiron or muscle-splitting incision for appendectomy. IMJ Ill Med J. 1969;135(3):287–8, passim.
14. Kelly HA, Hurdon E. The vermiform appendix and its diseases. Philadelphia: W.B. Saunders and Company; 1905.
15. Morse LJ, Rader MJ. Acute appendicitis: a twenty-year clinical survey. Ann Surg. 1940;111(2):213–29.
16. Ladd WE. Immediate or deferred surgery for general peritonitis associated with appendicitis in children. N Engl J Med. 1938;219(10):329–33.
17. Tan SY, Tatsumura Y. Alexander Fleming (1881–1955): discoverer of penicillin. Singap Med J. 2015;56(7):366–7.
18. Aycock TB, Farris EM. Appendicitis: the possible effects of sulfonamides on mortality. Ann Surg. 1945;121(5):710–7.
19. Ravitch MM. Appendicitis. Pediatrics. 1982;70(3):414–9.
20. Gross RE, Ladd WE. The surgery of infancy and childhood. Its principles and techniques. Philadelphia/London: W.B. Saunders Co; 1953. p. 112.
21. Semm K. Endoscopic appendectomy. Endoscopy. 1983;15(2):59–64.
22. Gongidi P, Bellah RD. Ultrasound of the pediatric appendix. Pediatr Radiol. 2017;47(9):1091–100.
23. Coward S, Kareemi H, Clement F, Zimmer S, Dixon E, Ball CG, et al. Incidence of appendicitis over time: a comparative analysis of an administrative healthcare database and a pathology-proven appendicitis registry. PLoS One. 2016;11(11):e0165161.
24. Lee SL, Ho HS. Acute appendicitis: is there a difference between children and adults? Am Surg. 2006;72(5):409–13.
25. Hawk JC Jr, Becker WF, Lehman EP. Acute appendicitis. III. Analysis of 1003 cases. Ann Surg. 1950;132(4):729–45.
26. Addiss DG, Shaffer N, Fowler BS, Tauxe RV. The epidemiology of appendicitis and appendectomy in the United States. Am J Epidemiol. 1990;132(5):910–25.
27. Peltokallio P, Tykka H. Evolution of the age distribution and mortality of acute appendicitis. Arch Surg. 1981;116(2):153–6.
28. Richardson MH. Appendicitis. Trans Am Surg Assoc. 1899;17:72.
29. Chau DB, Ciullo SS, Watson-Smith D, Chun TH, Kurkchubasche AG, Luks FI. Patient-centered outcomes research in appendicitis in children: bridging the knowledge gap. J Pediatr Surg. 2016;51(1):117–21.

Defining the Disease: Uncomplicated Versus Complicated Appendicitis

2

Christie Buonpane and Seth Goldstein

Case Example
An 11-year-old girl is undergoing a laparoscopic appendectomy. Intraoperatively the surgeon notes a fibrinous exudate on the appendix and murky fluid in the pelvis but not frank hole in the appendix. Do these intraoperative findings provide sufficient detail to define this as a case of uncomplicated or complicated appendicitis? And will this affect postoperative management?

Introduction

The nomenclature used to describe appendicitis has been debated for decades. Many postulate that appendicitis has a temporal progression, starting with simple uncomplicated disease, which, left untreated, will progress to perforation [1]. Others suggest that perforated and non-perforated appendicitis have different pathophysiology, and many episodes of uncomplicated appendicitis will spontaneously resolve without development of perforation [2]. Clinical treatment pathways and patient outcomes differ between uncomplicated and complicated appendicitis; however, a lack of consensus or standardization for the definition currently exists.

Terminologies such as "uncomplicated versus complicated," "non-perforated versus perforated," and "simple versus complex" are often used to describe appendicitis (Fig. 2.1). The reported incidence of complicated appendicitis ranges dramatically from 20% to 76%, which is likely due to the lack of standardization in the definition [3]. The strictest definition of complicated appendicitis only includes patients with a visible hole in the appendix or fecalith in the abdomen [4, 5].

C. Buonpane (✉) · S. Goldstein
Ann & Robert H. Lurie Children's Hospital of Chicago, Chicago, IL, USA

Northwestern University, Chicago, IL, USA
e-mail: Cbuonpane@luriechildrens.org

© Springer Nature Switzerland AG 2019
C. J. Hunter (ed.), *Controversies in Pediatric Appendicitis*,
https://doi.org/10.1007/978-3-030-15006-8_2

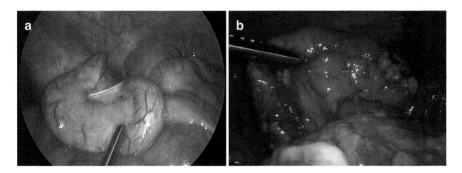

Fig. 2.1 (**a**) Intraoperative view of uncomplicated appendicitis. The appendix appears enlarged and hyperemic. (**b**) Intraoperative view of complicated appendicitis. Two focal areas of perforation can be seen, both at the base and tip of the appendix

Table 2.1 A summary of the various definitions of complicated appendicitis utilized in the current literature

Definitions of complicated appendicitis	
Fallon et al. [7] Retrospective review	"Gangrenous appendicitis has an ischemic, discolored wall without evidence of a hole or frank pus. Perforated appendicitis includes those with a hole, frank pus, or a fecalith"
	"Acute necrotizing/gangrenous appendicitis is acute appendicitis + any focus of transmural myonecrosis of the muscularis propria with an intact serosa. Perforations can be gross or microscopic"
Li et al. [8] Systematic review	"Gangrenous appendicitis, perforated appendix without phlegmon or abscess, or perforated appendicitis with phlegmon or abscess"
Yau et al. [9] Retrospective review	"Operative findings of gangrenous or perforated appendix with or without abscess formation"
Vaos et al. [10] Meta-analysis	"Operative findings of a perforated appendix according to the surgeon's diagnosis, or a periappendicular abscess or phlegmon, or appendiceal perforation confirmed in pathology report"
Varadhan et al. [11] Meta-analysis	"Local or contained perforation with an appendicular abscess or mass"
Athanasiou et al. [12] Systematic review Meta-analysis	"Histologically or intraoperatively diagnosed perforated appendix with or without free or localised pus or gangrenous appendix"
Fraser et al. [13] Prospective randomized trial	"Perforation was defined as an identifiable hole in the appendix or a fecalith in the abdomen"

All other patients, including a broad spectrum of disease, would be categorized as uncomplicated. Other classification systems consider suppurative/phlegmonous findings as uncomplicated and necrotic/gangrenous/perforated/ abscess as complicated [6]. A wide variability exists in the definitions utilized in appendicitis studies. Table 2.1 provides examples of various definitions of complicated appendicitis used in the literature [7–13].

The postoperative clinical pathway, patient outcomes, and morbidity differ dramatically between uncomplicated and complicated appendicitis [7]. Appropriate categorization of patients with complicated appendicitis is important in order to employ the proper treatment pathway and reduce the risk of postoperative abscess formation and other associated complications. St. Peter et al. demonstrated that a strict definition of complicated appendicitis (visible hole in the appendix or a fecalith in the abdomen) is effective in identifying patients at risk for postoperative abscess formation and would avoid overtreatment in patients with purulent or gangrenous appendicitis [4]. Analysis of patients with gangrenous appendicitis showed that outcomes and morbidity rates resemble those of simple appendicitis and that treatment should follow the uncomplicated clinical pathway [14, 15]. Others believe that patients with gangrenous appendicitis should be treated as complicated disease [6]. Standardization of these terms is crucial in order to reliably study patient outcomes in appendicitis and to avoid overtreatment of patients and prolonged hospital stays.

The definition of uncomplicated versus complicated appendicitis may be chosen from intraoperative findings, histopathology results, or a combination of both. However, postoperative clinical management is often dictated by intraoperative findings and employed prior to histopathology results. Intraoperative classification of appendicitis by the operating surgeon is often specific to the individual and can vary within a department and between institutions. Van den Boom et al. found considerable inter-observer variability exists in the intraoperative classification of appendicitis [16]. Additionally, there is an 8–10% discrepancy between intraoperative classification and the histopathologic diagnosis [7]. Often, intraoperative findings dictate postoperative management, and pathology results are used for official ICD-9 billing diagnoses. The application of retrospective review findings in clinical practice is complicated by these discrepancies.

Conclusion

Although appendicitis has been recognized for over a century, a lack of standardization in defining the disease still exists today. The definition of uncomplicated versus complicated appendicitis is crucial due to its impact on clinical decision making and patient outcomes. Proper definition of the disease could have direct effects on patient quality of care, complication rates, hospital costs, and length of stay. In the case example, fibrinous exudate and murky fluid are found intraoperatively, but without a frank hole in the appendix. In our opinion, this patient should be classified as having uncomplicated appendicitis, and postoperative care should follow the uncomplicated clinical pathway. This will avoid overtreatment with prolonged antibiotics and shorten hospital length of stay without increasing the risk of postoperative abscess formation or other complications [4, 17].

In addition to effects on patient quality of care and outcomes, the strict categorization of uncomplicated and complicated appendicitis has a vast effect on the ability of different institutions to compare results and study appendicitis outcomes. Due to the different interpretations and definitions of appendicitis, data published may be unreliable because of the ill-defined denominator [4]. In order to properly study the disease and allow for institutions to compare results in a meaningful way, standardization of the definition must exist.

Clinical Pearls

- A lack of standardization in the definition of appendicitis still exists today.
- Treatment pathways differ for uncomplicated and complicated appendicitis.
- Appropriate categorization of appendicitis can have direct effects on patient quality of care and outcomes.

References

1. Andersson RE. The natural history and traditional management of appendicitis revisited: spontaneous resolution and predominance of prehospital perforations imply that a correct diagnosis is more important than an early diagnosis. World J Surg. 2007;31(1):86–92.
2. Atema JJ, van Rossem CC, Leeuwenburgh MM, Stoker J, Boermeester MA. Scoring system to distinguish uncomplicated from complicated acute appendicitis. Br J Surg. 2015;102(8):979–90.
3. Newman K, Ponsky T, Kittle K, Dyk L, Throop C, Gieseker K, et al. Appendicitis 2000: variability in practice, outcomes, and resource utilization at thirty pediatric hospitals. J Pediatr Surg. 2003;38(3):372–9; discussion 9.
4. St Peter SD, Sharp SW, Holcomb GW 3rd, Ostlie DJ. An evidence-based definition for perforated appendicitis derived from a prospective randomized trial. J Pediatr Surg. 2008;43(12):2242–5.
5. Rentea RM, St Peter SD. Pediatric appendicitis. Surg Clin North Am. 2017;97(1):93–112.
6. Bhangu A, Soreide K, Di Saverio S, Assarsson JH, Drake FT. Acute appendicitis: modern understanding of pathogenesis, diagnosis, and management. Lancet. 2015;386(10000):1278–87.
7. Fallon SC, Kim ME, Hallmark CA, Carpenter JL, Eldin KW, Lopez ME, et al. Correlating surgical and pathological diagnoses in pediatric appendicitis. J Pediatr Surg. 2015;50(4):638–41.
8. Li Z, Zhao L, Cheng Y, Cheng N, Deng Y. Abdominal drainage to prevent intra-peritoneal abscess after open appendectomy for complicated appendicitis. Cochrane Database Syst Rev. 2018;5:CD010168.
9. Yau KK, Siu WT, Tang CN, Yang GP, Li MK. Laparoscopic versus open appendectomy for complicated appendicitis. J Am Coll Surg. 2007;205(1):60–5.
10. Vaos G, Dimopoulou A, Gkioka E, Zavras N. Immediate surgery or conservative treatment for complicated acute appendicitis in children? A meta-analysis. J Pediatr Surg. 2018 Jul 27. pii: S0022–3468(18)30478–0. https://doi.org/10.1016/j.jpedsurg.2018.07.017. [Epub ahead of print].
11. Varadhan KK, Neal KR, Lobo DN. Safety and efficacy of antibiotics compared with appendicectomy for treatment of uncomplicated acute appendicitis: meta-analysis of randomised controlled trials. BMJ. 2012;344:e2156.
12. Athanasiou C, Lockwood S, Markides GA. Systematic review and meta-analysis of laparoscopic versus open appendicectomy in adults with complicated appendicitis: an update of the literature. World J Surg. 2017;41(12):3083–99.
13. Fraser JD, Aguayo P, Leys CM, Keckler SJ, Newland JG, Sharp SW, et al. A complete course of intravenous antibiotics vs a combination of intravenous and oral antibiotics

for perforated appendicitis in children: a prospective, randomized trial. J Pediatr Surg. 2010;45(6):1198–202.

14. Emil S, Laberge JM, Mikhail P, Baican L, Flageole H, Nguyen L, et al. Appendicitis in children: a ten-year update of therapeutic recommendations. J Pediatr Surg. 2003;38(2):236–42.

15. Shbat L, Emil S, Elkady S, Baird R, Laberge JM, Puligandla P, et al. Benefits of an abridged antibiotic protocol for treatment of gangrenous appendicitis. J Pediatr Surg. 2014;49(12):1723–5.

16. van den Boom AL, de Wijkerslooth EML, Mauff KAL, Dawson I, van Rossem CC, Toorenvliet BR, et al. Interobserver variability in the classification of appendicitis during laparoscopy. Br J Surg. 2018;105(8):1014–9.

17. Emil S, Gaied F, Lo A, Laberge JM, Puligandla P, Shaw K, et al. Gangrenous appendicitis in children: a prospective evaluation of definition, bacteriology, histopathology, and outcomes. J Surg Res. 2012;177(1):123–6.

Making the Diagnosis: The Use of Clinical Features and Scoring Systems

3

Young Mee Choi and Steven Moulton

Case Example

An 8-year-old girl presents to the emergency department (ED) with a 2-day history of right lower quadrant (RLQ) abdominal pain. She had one episode of emesis and diarrhea the night before and decreased oral intake for the past 24 hours. She is otherwise a healthy child. She is afebrile with stable vital signs. Her abdominal examination is unremarkable except for mild tenderness on the right side without rebound tenderness or guarding. Blood work and ultrasound are ordered due to suspicion for acute appendicitis (AA). Results show an elevated white blood cell count of 13,000/μL without neutrophilia, and the ultrasound findings are equivocal. The ED physician calls for a surgical consult. What are the next steps in determining whether or not this child has AA?

Introduction

Abdominal pain is a common complaint among various childhood illnesses, ranging from nonsurgical conditions such as mesenteric adenitis or constipation to surgical conditions such as AA and bowel obstruction. Of these, AA is the most common surgical cause of abdominal pain but comprises of only 1–8% of children with abdominal pain seeking medical care [1, 2]. Prompt recognition of children with suspected AA and early intervention can avoid delays in diagnosis and lower the

Y. M. Choi
Children's Hospital Colorado, Aurora, CO, USA

Rutgers New Jersey Medical School, Newark, NJ, USA

S. Moulton (✉)
Children's Hospital Colorado, Aurora, CO, USA

University of Colorado School of Medicine, Aurora, CO, USA
e-mail: Steven.Moulton@childrenscolorado.org

© Springer Nature Switzerland AG 2019
C. J. Hunter (ed.), *Controversies in Pediatric Appendicitis*,
https://doi.org/10.1007/978-3-030-15006-8_3

risks of complications such as perforation and abscess formation [3]. Modern practice relies heavily on imaging studies to diagnose AA. As a result, many children who are at low risk for AA and could be screened with a scoring system are instead imaged, leading to unnecessary radiation exposure and increased healthcare costs. Although the use of ultrasound is increasing while the use of computed tomography (CT) is decreasing, the overall use of imaging studies still remains high [4]. Accurate clinical assessment in combination with a valid scoring system has the potential to limit the overuse of diagnostic imaging, hospital expenditures, and the number of false-positives or indeterminate study results and reduce unnecessary surgical procedures.

History and Physical Examination

Clinicians evaluating children with abdominal pain should be knowledgeable about the varying presentations of AA in different age groups. The history is usually obtained from parents or caregivers of infants and preadolescent children, who are unable to verbalize their symptoms. Abdominal pain is the most common complaint in a child with AA, and its characteristics, including the duration, severity, and alleviating and exacerbating factors, should be explored. The classic symptoms of periumbilical pain and nausea, followed by migration of the pain to the RLQ, and subsequent vomiting and fever may be difficult to elicit from preadolescent children. Moreover, the typical sequence of events describing the classic symptoms of appendicitis is thought to be present in less than 50% of children with AA [5, 6]. Typical symptoms such as migration of pain, RLQ pain, and anorexia are absent in 32–50% of children [7–9], and the absence of these symptoms does not rule out AA.

The duration of abdominal pain can point to whether it is an acute or chronic pathology, and exacerbating factors such as jumping or coughing may indicate peritoneal inflammation. The associated symptoms and review of systems can provide insight to the underlying disease process. For example, urinary symptoms may be present in AA but can also indicate a urinary tract infection, which is common in children. Bilious vomiting may suggest malrotation with small bowel obstruction or intussusception, and a bloody stool may suggest intussusception or Meckel's diverticulum.

Prior to the physical examination, it is important to ensure that the child receives adequate analgesia to reduce the level of anxiety and distress. Opioid administration does not interfere with the accuracy of the diagnosis and therefore should not be withheld due to concerns of masking signs or symptoms [10]. In general, a child presenting with AA will have RLQ tenderness or even signs of localized or generalized peritonitis, with involuntary guarding and rebound tenderness. Right lower quadrant tenderness and pain on movement (coughing or hopping) have the highest sensitivity for AA [7]. Other commonly described clinical signs of AA include tenderness at McBurney's point (one-third of the distance from the anterior superior iliac spine to the umbilicus), Rovsing sign (pain in the right lower quadrant on palpation of the left side), obturator sign (pain on flexion and internal rotation of the right hip, suggestive of an inflamed appendix in the pelvis), and iliopsoas sign (pain on extension of the right hip, suggestive of retrocecal appendicitis). Unfortunately, many of these signs are difficult to elicit in a young, uncooperative child. Rovsing sign was found to be the physical exam finding most suggestive of AA in a large meta-analysis [6], but it is present in only 32% of children with AA [9], which reduces its applicability.

An assessment of the probability of perforated AA can guide treatment and the expected hospital course. The age of the child is important when assessing the probability of perforated AA, since younger age is associated with a higher risk of perforated AA. One study reported that perforation was present in 100% of children ≤1 year of age, 93% of children aged 2 years, and 69% of children aged 5 years [7, 11]. The duration of symptoms is also significantly associated with the severity of AA [12]. In the original study by Alvarado, children with simple AA presented with a mean of 1.2 days of symptoms, whereas those with complicated AA with an abscess had a mean of 9.3 days of symptoms [12]. Differentiating perforated from nonperforated AA may be difficult on physical examination, but children with perforated AA will generally appear ill and have higher temperatures than those with nonperforated AA [13].

Special Considerations

Neonates
Neonatal AA is rare. Fewer than 50 cases have been reported in the last 30 years in the literature, and the mortality rate is reported to be as high as 28% [14, 15]. It affects preterm newborns as well as full-term infants [14, 16], and the most common presenting sign is abdominal distension, present in 75% of reported cases [14]. Less common signs and symptoms include vomiting, irritability, restlessness, anorexia, temperature instability, and abdominal tenderness [15]. Neonatal AA can be mistaken for necrotizing enterocolitis, due to the nonspecific but similar presenting clinical picture, and therefore it is often managed non-operatively, leading to a delay in diagnosis and a lost opportunity for appropriate surgical intervention. It is important, therefore, to be aware and keep AA in the differential when evaluating a newborn with abdominal distension and sepsis, without clear signs of necrotizing enterocolitis.

Infants (2 Years or Younger)
Acute appendicitis is uncommon in this age group, and a large proportion of children present with perforated AA. The most common symptoms in this age group are vomiting (85–90%), abdominal pain (35–77%), diarrhea (18–46%), and fever (40–60%) [17]. Less common symptoms such as abdominal distention (30–52%) or rigidity (23%) can help guide clinicians to an intra-abdominal process. Vomiting and fever, however, can mimic the symptoms of other common childhood illnesses, such as gastroenteritis or an upper respiratory tract infection. The presence of other nonspecific symptoms such as irritability (35–40%), lethargy (40%), and

right hip pain or stiffness (3–23%) can further delay the diagnosis of AA in this age group [17].

Preadolescent (3–11 years)

Emesis, in addition to the classic symptoms of AA, is seen in up to 66% of preadolescent children with AA; however, emesis is equally common in children with abdominal pain due to other causes, yielding low specificity. Similarly, fever, defined as a temperature ≥38 °C, is a common finding in children with abdominal pain, affecting 47% of those with AA versus 53% of those without AA [7], although this sign may indicate perforation in the setting of AA [8].

Missed AA occurs more frequently in younger children compared to those who are older and correctly diagnosed at initial presentation (mean age 5 years vs 8 years), due to the high incidence of atypical symptoms in the age group ≤5 years old [18]. Symptoms that are atypical of AA include diarrhea, irritability, lethargy, and vomiting before the onset of abdominal pain. Other atypical symptoms such as dysuria, constipation, and respiratory tract symptoms may lead the clinician to other diagnoses such as urinary or respiratory tract infection [18], resulting in a delayed or missed diagnosis.

Adolescent (12–18 years)

Clinicians can generally obtain a more reliable history and physical examination from the adolescent population. Adolescents are likely to present in a manner similar to adults with the classic symptoms of AA. The overall incidence of AA is higher in this age group, but the rate of perforation is lower compared to younger age groups, presumably due to earlier diagnosis. Obtaining menstrual and sexual history from female patients of childbearing age is important, because gynecologic conditions such as ovarian torsion, pelvic inflammatory disease, and ectopic pregnancy can mimic the clinical presentation of AA.

The Role of Scoring Systems in the Management of Appendicitis

Efforts to standardiaze the work up and management of patients with suspected AA have led clinicians to create scoring systems, which categorize patients into different risk strata to better guide management. These systems, when properly used, can reduce the number and types of imaging studies employed when evaluating a child with abdominal pain. They are particularly useful when evaluating children with a low to intermediate likelihood of AA.

It is worthwhile to mention the key elements of scoring systems. Scoring systems are regression-based, with different numerical weights given to the predictor variables. The models undergo validation studies in various study populations prior to being used in clinical practice. Of the statistical performance characteristics of a scoring system, perhaps the most important and relevant one to a surgeon is the positive predictive value (PPV), which relates to the ability to identify children with

Table 3.1 Alvarado score and pediatric appendicitis score

	Alvarado score		Pediatric appendicitis score (PAS)	
Symptoms	Migration of pain	1	Migration of pain	1
	Anorexia	1	Anorexia	1
	Nausea/emesis	1	Nausea/emesis	1
Signs	Right lower quadrant tenderness	2	Right lower quadrant tenderness	2
	Rebound pain	1	Cough/hopping/percussion tenderness in the right lower quadrant	2
	Elevation in temperature (≥37 °C)	1	Elevation in temperature (≥38 °C)	1
Laboratory	Leukocytes ≥10,000/µL	2	Leukocytes ≥10,000/µL	1
	Polymorphonuclear neutrophilia ≥75%	1	Polymorphonuclear neutrophilia ≥75%	1
	Total	10	Total	10

AA in the high-risk group and therefore determine the rate of negative appendectomies [19]. Negative predictive value (NPV) would impact the percentage of children who are misdiagnosed and therefore suffer from missed AA, which can be detrimental. Both the PPV and NPV are affected by the prevalence of the disease in a population. A scoring system with high sensitivity helps clinicians be certain that children with AA would be given high scores and correctly diagnosed, and high specificity increases confidence that children without AA would be given low scores and therefore excluded. A careful balance needs to be met to find a cutoff point to optimize the performance statistics through rigorous validation studies.

To date, the *Alvarado score* and the *pediatric appendicitis score (PAS)* are the most widely studied scoring systems in the pediatric literature [20]. The Alvarado score was developed based on pediatric and adult data [12] and has subsequently been validated in multiple pediatric studies. The PAS was developed specifically for children [21]. Both scoring systems are based on eight predictive factors, consisting of symptoms, signs, and two laboratory values (Table 3.1). An Alvarado score of 1–4 represents low probability of AA, and most of these patients can be discharged. An Alvarado score of 5–6 is considered intermediate risk, and these patients need further workup or in-hospital observation. A score of 7–8 is considered probable AA, and 9–10 is considered high likelihood of AA. The latter two groups typically undergo surgical intervention. The PAS originally defined two risk categories: 1–5 as low probability of AA and 6–10 as high probability AA, the latter requiring surgical intervention. There remains ongoing debate as to what the ideal cutoff value should be to achieve the highest accuracy of diagnosing AA for both scoring systems. Cutoff values of 6 and 7 for both scores have been suggested [22, 23], but the original cutoff values are still being used.

Studies comparing the two scoring systems generally agree that the scores provide useful diagnostic information when evaluating children with suspected AA without significant differences between the two, although neither provides a PPV that is high enough to be used as the single method for the diagnosis of AA and determining the need for surgery [19, 22]. A systematic review suggests that the

Alvarado score has higher sensitivity than the PAS, but the two scoring systems have similar specificities [20].

The Alvarado score together with positive ultrasound findings (compressibility, presence of free fluid, tenderness, hyperemia, and size of the appendix) has been shown to increase the sensitivity (98%) and specificity (82%) of diagnosing AA in adults [24]. However, this study had a high incidence of non-visualization of the appendix on ultrasound (37%) with 59% of patients requiring further imaging with CT or MRI. While this approach of combining a scoring system with imaging findings was shown to increase diagnostic accuracy, it would require that all children with suspected AA undergo ultrasound. The combination of a scoring system with ultrasound findings may be useful in the intermediate group (e.g., Alvarado score 5–6), and the risks and benefits of using imaging versus observation alone should be further explored.

The Appendicitis Inflammatory Response (AIR) score incorporates signs and symptoms as well as C-reactive protein (CRP) [25]. It grades the clinical features and laboratory values according to the severity of each element, rather than as dichotomous variables. It was primarily developed on adult data but later validated in children. An AIR score of 0–4 represents low probability of AA; a score of 5–8 identifies an indeterminate group requiring in-hospital observation with additional imaging or diagnostic laparoscopy; a score of 9–12 represents high probability of AA. The AIR score can be easily applied in children because it does not involve subjective signs such as nausea and migration of pain. The one drawback to its use is the need to draw a CRP level, which may not be readily available in some hospitals. One study found that implementation of the AIR score significantly reduced the incidence of negative explorations (3.2% to 1.6%) and hospital admissions compared to a historic cohort (from 43% to 30%) [26]. In the same study, the proportion of children undergoing imaging also significantly decreased in the high-risk group (53% to 38.5%), without significant differences in the rate of negative explorations, admissions, and readmissions to the hospital [27]. When children in the intermediate group were randomized to observation or imaging, those randomized to imaging were more frequently diagnosed with AA, without significant differences in readmission or missed appendicitis rates between the two groups.

The *appendicitis score* was derived from 127 children ages 4–15 years old. The score consists of male gender (2 points); intensity of pain (2 for severe pain); relocation of pain (4 points); vomiting (2 points); pain in the RLQ (4 points); fever ≥37.5 °C (3 points); guarding (4 points); absent, tinkling, or high-pitched bowel sounds (4 points); and rebound tenderness (7 points) giving a maximum of 32 points [28]. Scores of 21 or more indicate high probability of AA; scores of 15 or less indicate low probability of AA. Scores from 16 to 20 represent intermediate probability. The authors recommend appendectomy in those with RLQ pain, rebound, or guarding even if the score is 15 or less due to the high likelihood of AA in children with these symptoms. When children were randomized to the appendicitis-score or a no-score group in a different prospective cohort of 126 children, the authors found a significantly higher negative appendectomy rate in the no-score group (29% vs. 17%, $p = 0.05$) and higher diagnostic accuracy in the appendicitis-score group (92%

vs. 80% $p = 0.04$), without significant differences in the rate of missed AA between the two groups [29].

Lastly, the *pediatric appendicitis risk calculator (pARC)* outputs a predicted risk of AA on a continuous scale and is derived from a sample of 2423 children ages 5–18 years old [30]. The predicted risk is categorized into low- (predicted risk of 0–14%), intermediate- (15–84%), and high-risk groups ($\geq$85%). Variables in the calculator include male gender, age groups, duration of pain, pain with walking, migration of pain to the RLQ, maximal tenderness in RLQ, abdominal guarding, and ANC value. It has similar diagnostic accuracy as the PAS, but requires sophisticated calculations, which can be built into a program to make it user-friendly. It has yet to be validated in different study populations.

This is not an exhaustive list of the available appendicitis scoring systems, but rather a brief review of those most relevant to children. Scoring systems have the potential to standardize care and reduce unnecessary admissions and diagnostic studies, but remain underutilized in clinical settings. Their utilization may be improved with a scoring system that is built into the hospital electronic medical charting system to lessen the burden on the clinical staff and make it easier to use. As some of the studies show, there are demonstrable benefits to the routine use of a scoring system, and children with indeterminate study results may benefit from careful observation rather than routine imaging studies [27, 29]. There are limitations to using scoring systems when diagnosing AA in children. One limitation is that some of the history elements of a scoring system are not easily assessable in young and nonverbal children. Another limitation is that the examination findings may be clinician-dependent, even though most scoring systems use relatively simple examination findings such as RLQ tenderness or rebound tenderness. Lastly, the widespread use of ultrasound may avert clinicians from using scoring systems to determine the need for imaging studies.

Conclusion

More prospective studies are needed to test the efficacy of scoring systems at reducing hospital costs associated with overutilization of diagnostic studies, misdiagnosis or delay in diagnosis of AA, and negative appendectomies. Importantly, emerging technologies that estimate severity of illness in conditions such as appendicitis may complement and increase the accuracy of current scoring systems [31].

Clinical Pearls

- The Alvarado score and pediatric appendicitis score are the most widely studied scoring systems for acute appendicitis in children.
- Scoring systems stratify children into low, intermediate, and high probability groups.
- Scoring systems have the potential to reduce the rate of imaging studies, unnecessary hospital admissions, and negative appendectomies.

- Prospective trials are needed to compare and assess the effectiveness of scoring systems at expediting the diagnosis of acute appendicitis and reducing unnecessary interventions.

References

1. Reynolds SL, Jaffe DM. Diagnosing abdominal pain in a pediatric emergency department. Pediatr Emerg Care. 1992;8(3):126–8.
2. Scholer SJ, Pituch K, Orr DP, Dittus RS. Clinical outcomes of children with acute abdominal pain. Pediatrics. 1996;98(4 Pt 1):680–5.
3. Papandria D, Goldstein SD, Rhee D, Salazar JH, Arlikar J, Gorgy A, et al. Risk of perforation increases with delay in recognition and surgery for acute appendicitis. J Surg Res. 2013;184(2):723–9.
4. Bachur RG, Levy JA, Callahan MJ, Rangel SJ, Monuteaux MC. Effect of reduction in the use of computed tomography on clinical outcomes of appendicitis. JAMA Pediatr. 2015;169(8):755–60.
5. Bundy DG, Byerley JS, Liles EA, Perrin EM, Katznelson J, Rice HE. Does this child have appendicitis? JAMA. 2007;298(4):438–51.
6. Benabbas R, Hanna M, Shah J, Sinert R. Diagnostic accuracy of history, physical examination, laboratory tests, and point-of-care ultrasound for pediatric acute appendicitis in the emergency department: a systematic review and meta-analysis. Acad Emerg Med. 2017;24(5):523–51.
7. Colvin JM, Bachur R, Kharbanda A. The presentation of appendicitis in preadolescent children. Pediatr Emerg Care. 2007;23(12):849–55.
8. Sakellaris G, Tilemis S, Charissis G. Acute appendicitis in preschool-age children. Eur J Pediatr. 2005;164(2):80–3.
9. Becker T, Kharbanda A, Bachur R. Atypical clinical features of pediatric appendicitis. Acad Emerg Med. 2007;14(2):124–9.
10. Bailey B, Bergeron S, Gravel J, Bussieres JF, Bensoussan A. Efficacy and impact of intravenous morphine before surgical consultation in children with right lower quadrant pain suggestive of appendicitis: a randomized controlled trial. Ann Emerg Med. 2007;50(4):371–8.
11. Nance ML, Adamson WT, Hedrick HL. Appendicitis in the young child: a continuing diagnostic challenge. Pediatr Emerg Care. 2000;16(3):160–2.
12. Alvarado A. A practical score for the early diagnosis of acute appendicitis. Ann Emerg Med. 1986;15(5):557–64.
13. van den Bogaard VA, Euser SM, van der Ploeg T, de Korte N, Sanders DG, de Winter D, et al. Diagnosing perforated appendicitis in pediatric patients: a new model. J Pediatr Surg. 2016;51(3):444–8.
14. Schwartz KL, Gilad E, Sigalet D, Yu W, Wong AL. Neonatal acute appendicitis: a proposed algorithm for timely diagnosis. J Pediatr Surg. 2011;46(11):2060–4.
15. Karaman A, Cavusoglu YH, Karaman I, Cakmak O. Seven cases of neonatal appendicitis with a review of the English language literature of the last century. Pediatr Surg Int. 2003;19(11):707–9.
16. Jancelewicz T, Kim G, Miniati D. Neonatal appendicitis: a new look at an old zebra. J Pediatr Surg. 2008;43(10):e1–5.
17. Rothrock SG, Pagane J. Acute appendicitis in children: emergency department diagnosis and management. Ann Emerg Med. 2000;36(1):39–51.
18. Rothrock SG, Skeoch G, Rush JJ, Johnson NE. Clinical features of misdiagnosed appendicitis in children. Ann Emerg Med. 1991;20(1):45–50.
19. Schneider C, Kharbanda A, Bachur R. Evaluating appendicitis scoring systems using a prospective pediatric cohort. Ann Emerg Med. 2007;49(6):778–84, 784.e1

20. Ebell MH, Shinholser J. What are the most clinically useful cutoffs for the Alvarado and pediatric appendicitis scores? A systematic review. Ann Emerg Med. 2014;64(4):365–72.e2.
21. Samuel M. Pediatric appendicitis score. J Pediatr Surg. 2002;37(6):877–81.
22. Escriba A, Gamell AM, Fernandez Y, Quintilla JM, Cubells CL. Prospective validation of two systems of classification for the diagnosis of acute appendicitis. Pediatr Emerg Care. 2011;27(3):165–9.
23. Pogorelic Z, Rak S, Mrklic I, Juric I. Prospective validation of Alvarado score and pediatric appendicitis score for the diagnosis of acute appendicitis in children. Pediatr Emerg Care. 2015;31(3):164–8.
24. Reddy SB, Kelleher M, Bokhari SAJ, Davis KA, Schuster KM. A highly sensitive and specific combined clinical and sonographic score to diagnose appendicitis. J Trauma Acute Care Surg. 2017;83(4):643–9.
25. Andersson M, Andersson RE. The appendicitis inflammatory response score: a tool for the diagnosis of acute appendicitis that outperforms the Alvarado score. World J Surg. 2008;32(8):1843–9.
26. Macco S, Vrouenraets BC, de Castro SM. Evaluation of scoring systems in predicting acute appendicitis in children. Surgery. 2016;160(6):1599–604.
27. Andersson M, Kolodziej B, Andersson RE, Group SS. Randomized clinical trial of appendicitis inflammatory response score-based management of patients with suspected appendicitis. Br J Surg. 2017;104(11):1451–61.
28. Lintula H, Pesonen E, Kokki H, Vanamo K, Eskelinen M. A diagnostic score for children with suspected appendicitis. Langenbeck's Arch Surg. 2005;390(2):164–70.
29. Lintula H, Kokki H, Kettunen R, Eskelinen M. Appendicitis score for children with suspected appendicitis. A randomized clinical trial. Langenbeck's Arch Surg. 2009;394(6):999–1004.
30. Kharbanda AB, Vazquez-Benitez G, Ballard DW, Vinson DR, Chettipally UK, Kene MV, et al. Development and validation of a novel pediatric appendicitis risk calculator (pARC). Pediatrics. 2018;141(4). https://doi.org/10.1542/peds.2017-2699.
31. Choi YM, Leopold D, Campbell K, Mulligan J, Grudic GZ, Moulton SL. Noninvasive monitoring of physiologic compromise in acute appendicitis: new insight into an old disease. J Pediatr Surg. 2018;53(2):241–6.

The Role and Efficacy of Laboratories in the Diagnosis of Pediatric Appendicitis

4

Colin Martin and Raoud Marayati

Case Example

A 5-year-old is brought to her pediatrician's office because of abdominal pain and loss of appetite. On exam the pediatrician finds that the child has pain in her lower abdomen, but it is difficult to tell the precise location of the pain. The patient does not currently have a fever; however, the pediatrician is concerned that this patient has appendicitis. The child is referred to the emergency room, and the pediatrician suggests that laboratory testing may be helpful in making the diagnosis.

Introduction

Making the Diagnosis

Appendicitis is one of the most common pediatric surgical emergencies. Operative intervention, in the form of appendectomy, is the gold standard, and a delay in diagnosis of acute appendicitis may be associated with increased risk or perforation and further complications. Historically the negative appendectomy rate has been reported to be as high as 30% [1]. Despite complete clinical history and physical examination, early acute appendicitis is still difficult to diagnose in children. Clinical examination remains one of the most sensitive diagnostic methods of pediatric appendicitis. However, it has been shown to carry a low specificity and a low positive predictive value. Thus, relying on clinical signs alone may result in a much

C. Martin (✉)
Department of Surgery, Division of Pediatric Surgery, University of Alabama at Birmingham, Birmingham, AL, USA
e-mail: colin.martin@childrensal.org

R. Marayati
Department of Surgery, University of Alabama at Birmingham, Birmingham, AL, USA

© Springer Nature Switzerland AG 2019
C. J. Hunter (ed.), *Controversies in Pediatric Appendicitis*,
https://doi.org/10.1007/978-3-030-15006-8_4

higher negative appendectomy rate, and thus the analysis of key laboratory values may be helpful in the diagnostic workup. The role of various laboratory markers in the workup of possible acute appendicitis has been widely studied, and their use is a source of continued debate. Laboratory analysis is often included as an important adjunct in making the diagnosis of appendicitis. For example, the pneumonic *MANTRELS* (Migration of pain to the right lower quadrant, Anorexia, Nausea/vomiting, Tenderness in the right lower quadrant, Rebound pain, Elevation of temperature, Leukocytosis, Shift of white blood cell (WBC) count to the left) includes a WBC. Other scoring systems (discussed in more detail in other chapters) such as the Ohmann score can accurately identify patients at low, moderate, and high risk for appendicitis by mathematically combining clinical and laboratory findings. Although imaging is helpful to make the diagnosis, the use of laboratory tests and other point-of-care algorithms [2] aims to minimize radiation exposure with CT scanning as well as unnecessary surgery while maintaining a high sensitivity for identifying appendicitis.

The typical laboratory workup for a patient with possible appendicitis includes a white blood cell (WBC) count with differential and urinalysis. Other commonly used laboratory tests include acute-phase proteins such as C-reactive protein (CRP). In early stages of appendicitis, laboratory evaluation may be within the reference range, because the inflammation and infection have not yet become systemically detectable. It has been suggested that laboratory values increase in diagnostic value as the patient's duration of symptoms increases.

White Blood Cell (WBC) Count

The WBC count is the most often used test to support the diagnosis of acute appendicitis. It is elevated in 70–90% of patients with acute appendicitis. WBC also has a limited predictive value with acceptable sensitivity (80–92%) and low specificity (29–76%). A threshold WBC of 10,000/μL was associated with a likelihood ratio (LR) of 2.0, a 15% increase in the probability of having acute appendicitis in patients with an elevated WBC [3]. Increasing the threshold of WBC count did not improve likelihood ratios and caused a significant decline in sensitivity. Leukocyte response declines in children below 5 years of age, and WBC count may be normal in 8% of infants with proven acute appendicitis [4]. WBC count lacks the diagnostic accuracy to be used as a single laboratory marker for appendicitis. However, its utility increases significantly when combined with the presence of a left shift or an elevated CRP.

Differential

The presence of a left shift or more than 80% polymorphonuclear cells and bands on a cell differential in the setting of an elevated WBC has been shown to have significant predictive power. An immature granulocyte percentage (IG%) is an automated hematologic analysis that is more accurate automated differentials. An elevated IG% has shown to be more accurate than standard neutrophil measures in predicating pediatric sepsis. However Matthews et al. demonstrated that elevated IG% was not a significant predictor of appendicitis [5].

C-Reactive Protein

C-reactive protein (CRP) rises in its serum concentration 6 hours after inflammation until the peak is reached in approximately 48 hours. Yang et al. performed a prospective case control series to correlate the laboratory findings with the diagnosis and severity of appendicitis. They found that CRP correlated with the positive diagnosis of appendicitis and was significantly associated with perforation. In a meta-analysis CRP has been shown to have a medium sensitivity (53–88%) and specificity (46–82%) for appendicitis. Patients with WBC greater than 12,000/μL and CRP greater than 3 mg/dl were 7.75 times more likely to have appendicitis [6]. CRP levels are significantly higher in children with perforated appendicitis than in simple uncomplicated appendicitis. CRP may be used in combination with a WBC to enhance the diagnosis of appendicitis.

Mean Platelet Volume (MPV)

Mean platelet volume is acute phase reactant and a marker of platelet activation and inflammation. Several studies have been shown that correlate MPV to sepsis. Although not confirmed in in pediatric studies, MPV has been shown be a predictor of acute appendicitis [7].

Hyperbilirubinemia

An elevated bilirubin level is associated with acute appendicitis. It has an 88% and positive predictive value of 91% for simple acute appendicitis. Emmanuel et al. performed a large retrospective review and found that a bilirubin level greater that 1.0 mg/dl has strong correlation with acute appendicitis and was a better prediction of gangrenous and perforated appendicitis. Although this study was conducted in adult patients, they found that an elevated bilirubin was a better predictor of appendicitis than CRP or WBC [8].

Urinalysis (UA)

Irritation of the bladder or ureter by an inflamed appendix may result in few urinary WBCs. In addition, urinary RBCs can be found in patients with appendicitis with an overlying phlegmon or abscess lying adjacent to the ureter, typically fewer than 20 per high-power field. Ketonuria is suggestive of dehydration and can be seen in perforated appendicitis. None of these findings, however, are reliable enough to confirm or exclude the diagnosis of acute appendicitis.

Since acute appendicitis is associated with an acute-phase reaction, many studies have shown that cytokines and acute-phase proteins are activated and may serve as indicators of the severity of appendicitis.

Erythrocyte Sedimentation Rate (ESR)

An increased ESR level has been shown to correlate with the grade of inflammation. However, the method of detection is non-specific, time-consuming, and not widely recommended.

Interleukin 6 (IL-6)

IL-6 is an inducer of acute phase protein synthesis in human hepatocytes causing a wide response including fever, high WBC, and increased immune activity. It is also a non-specific marker of inflammation with a short half-life. Bacteria and lipopoly-saccharide (endotoxin) are known to cause an increase in the release of a number of cytokines including TNF-α, IL-1, and IL-6. Sack et al. showed that CRP and IL-6 correlated significantly with the severity of appendiceal inflammation, with significantly higher levels in gangrenous and perforated acute appendicitis [6]. Serum levels of IL-6 were shown to differentiate between the children with acute appendicitis with perforation and those without perforation [9].

Conclusions

In summary, laboratory results should be integrated within the complete diagnostic assessment of acute appendicitis. They provide the most valuable information when combined in discerning the necessity for operative intervention. Of note, acute appendicitis is very unlikely when leucocyte count, neutrophil percentage, and CRP level are simultaneously with normal limits [10].

Clinical Pearls

- Laboratory values may be normal in very early acute appendicitis.
- Combining laboratory values may increase their predictive value in making the diagnosis of appendicitis.
- No single laboratory value is definitive in the diagnosis of appendicitis.

References

1. Christian F, Christian GP. A simple scoring system to reduce the negative appendicectomy rate. Ann R Coll Surg Engl. 1992;74(4):281–5.
2. Ebell MH. Diagnosis of appendicitis: part II. Laboratory and imaging tests. Am Fam Physician. 2008;77(8):1153–5.
3. Bundy DG. Clinical prediction rule identifies children at low risk for appendicitis. J Pediatr. 2013;162(3):654–5.
4. Paajanen H, Mansikka A, Laato M, Kettunen J, Kostiainen S. Are serum inflammatory markers age dependent in acute appendicitis? J Am Coll Surg. 1997;184(3):303–8.
5. Mathews EK, Griffin RL, Mortellaro V, Beierle EA, Harmon CM, Chen MK, et al. Utility of immature granulocyte percentage in pediatric appendicitis. J Surg Res. 2014;190(1):230–4.
6. Kwan KY, Nager AL. Diagnosing pediatric appendicitis: usefulness of laboratory markers. Am J Emerg Med. 2010;28(9):1009–15.
7. Fan Z, Zhang Y, Pan J, Wang S. Acute appendicitis and mean platelet volume: a systemic review and meta-analysis. Ann Clin Lab Sci. 2017;47(6):768–72.
8. Emmanuel A, Murchan P, Wilson I, Balfe P. The value of hyperbilirubinaemia in the diagnosis of acute appendicitis. Ann R Coll Surg Engl. 2011;93(3):213–7.
9. Groselj-Grenc M, Repse S, Dolenc-Strazar Z, Hojker S, Derganc M. Interleukin-6 and lipopolysaccharide-binding protein in acute appendicitis in children. Scand J Clin Lab Invest. 2007;67(2):197–206.
10. Yang HR, Wang YC, Chung PK, Chen WK, Jeng LB, Chen RJ. Laboratory tests in patients with acute appendicitis. ANZ J Surg. 2006;76(1–2):71–4.

Diagnostic Imaging for Pediatric Appendicitis

5

Dalya M. Ferguson, K. Tinsley Anderson, and KuoJen Tsao

Case Example

An 11-year-old, 45 kg, female presents to a community emergency department with 8 hours of abdominal pain. The emergency physician requests surgical consultation in anticipation of possible transfer and reports that the patient has tenderness to palpation in the right lower quadrant, but is afebrile and has a normal white blood cell count. She would like to know if you would like imaging for this patient and, if so, what?

Introduction

Appendectomy is the most common urgent surgical procedure in children, with approximately 80,000 appendectomies performed annually in the United States [1]. Appendicitis was traditionally diagnosed clinically, based on history and physical exam, and surgeons accepted a 10–20% rate of finding a normal appendix at surgery (negative appendectomy) [2]. With improving technology, abdominal ultrasonography (U/S) gained popularity in the late 1980s [3]. As computed tomography (CT) became more ubiquitous, its use supplanted U/S [4]. Magnetic resonance imaging (MRI) use has increased slowly over the past few years as the harms of CT-associated radiation have been acknowledged and publicized. The increase in accuracy and availability of diagnostic imaging has resulted in a decrease in the negative appendectomy rate, from 20% to 2%, over the past three decades [2, 5]. Today, nearly 100% of pediatric patients undergo some type of imaging to establish a diagnosis of appendicitis; CT accounts for more than 50% of these studies [6]. The choice of

D. M. Ferguson · K. T. Anderson · K. Tsao (✉)
Center for Surgical Trials and Evidence-Based Practice, McGovern Medical School at The University of Texas Health Science Center at Houston, Houston, TX, USA
e-mail: KuoJen.Tsao@uth.tmc.edu

© Springer Nature Switzerland AG 2019
C. J. Hunter (ed.), *Controversies in Pediatric Appendicitis*,
https://doi.org/10.1007/978-3-030-15006-8_5

imaging modality is highly dependent on clinician decision-making, as well as local availability and practices.

The ideal diagnostic imaging modality would expeditiously and accurately diagnose appendicitis without exposing the patient to additional harms and would be cost-effective. Each modality has limitations, risks, and benefits, which should be considered based on the clinical scenario. Adjuncts to imaging, such as radiology report templates, clinical scoring systems, and standardized algorithms for patient evaluation, have enhanced the value of diagnostic studies. Moreover, individual modalities should be thought of in conjunction with other study types as well as contextual and patient-related factors. The following review describes the advantages and limitations of each modality, followed by a discussion of ways to enhance the diagnostic utility of various imaging strategies.

Literature Review

Ultrasonography

Graded compression U/S was first described for the diagnosis of appendicitis in 1986 [3]. The traditional criterion for diagnosis of appendicitis by U/S is an appendiceal maximal outer diameter (MOD) >6 mm. Searle et al. looked at normal appendiceal diameter by age and found that the appendiceal diameter does not increase significantly above age 3 [7]. A retrospective review by Goldin et al. found that using diagnostic criteria of MOD $\geq$7 mm or wall thickness >1.7 mm had a sensitivity of 99% and specificity of 95% [8]. Among published meta-analyses of the diagnostic accuracy of U/S, sensitivity ranges from 0.88 to 0.91 and specificity from 0.90 to 0.97 (Table 5.1) [9–12]. Figure 5.1 shows the imaging findings of appendicitis by U/S.

While MOD is a central component of U/S diagnosis of appendicitis, one criticism of U/S is the frequency of lack of visualization (full or partial) of the appendix, which occurs 18–75% of the time [19–21]. According to a multicenter prospective observational study by Mittal et al., U/S had a specificity of 97% and a sensitivity of 72.5% for the diagnosis of appendicitis in children ages 3–18 [22]. The primary reason for

Table 5.1 Ranges of sensitivity and specificity for different imaging modalities by source [9–18]

	Ultrasonography (U/S)	Computed tomography (CT)	Magnetic resonance imaging (MRI)
Test characteristics			
Sensitivity:			
Single studies	0.44–1.00	0.76–0.97	0.85–1.00
Meta-analyses	0.88–0.91	0.90–0.95	0.96–0.98
Specificity:			
Single studies	0.86–0.97	0.83–0.99	0.96–0.98
Meta-analyses	0.90–0.97	0.92–0.95	0.96–0.97

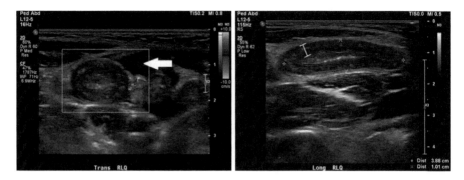

Fig. 5.1 Ultrasound positive for appendicitis. Transverse view (left) demonstrates periappendiceal free fluid (arrow). Longitudinal view (right) highlights appendiceal wall thickening, with a maximal outer diameter of 1.01 cm

the lower sensitivity was the frequency with which the appendix was not visualized. In cases where the appendix was visualized, the sensitivity was 97.9%, and the specificity was 91.7%. However, lack of visualization has a high negative predictive value for appendicitis [23]. The combination of lack of visualization and absence of secondary findings reduces the likelihood of appendicitis to less than 2% [24].

Secondary findings that may support the diagnosis of appendicitis include appendiceal wall thickness ≥3 mm, non-compressibility of the appendix, wall hyperemia on color Doppler, periappendiceal mesenteric fat stranding, presence of an appendicolith, free fluid, a periappendiceal hypoechoic halo indicative of appendiceal wall edema, lymphadenopathy, and abdominal tenderness during U/S examination. Published literature provides contradictory data on the diagnostic value of secondary signs for the diagnosis of appendicitis with U/S. Goldin et al. reported that incorporating secondary findings into diagnostic criteria did not increase the sensitivity or specificity of U/S [8]. Trout et al. found that periappendiceal fat stranding was the only secondary finding that was statistically significant in predicting the presence of appendicitis [25]. In one retrospective review of imaging in negative appendectomies, the most common U/S findings that misled radiologists were non-compressibility (56%) and sonographic tenderness (56%), followed by RLQ lymphadenopathy (50%) [26]. Nevertheless, the presence of secondary findings in the setting of a non-visualized appendix or the absence of secondary findings in the setting of a borderline MOD may increase diagnostic accuracy [20].

The primary limitation of U/S is its operator dependence. Techniques for improved appendix visualization have been reported, including standard supine scanning, followed by left posterior oblique scanning if the appendix is not visualized, and then "second-look" supine scanning [27]. Increased use of U/S, i.e., practice, is also associated with decreased non-visualization of the appendix and improved diagnostic accuracy [19]. Sensitivity is higher at centers with higher U/S utilization, and nondiagnostic U/S studies are more prevalent at community hospitals, where CT is more often employed as the first imaging test [22, 28].

Additionally, U/S is commonly thought to perform worse than other imaging modalities in overweight or obese patients [29–31]. Increased abdominal wall thickness and retrocecal location are associated with decreased rates of visualization in adult studies [32]. However, U/S has been shown to maintain its diagnostic utility in children regardless of patient body habitus [33]. Techniques to improve visualization in patients with a large body habitus include posterior manual compression and use of lower-frequency transducers [34].

Utilizing a standardized radiology report template that incorporates secondary signs has been shown to improve U/S diagnostic clarity. Nielsen et al. formulated a template that defined an abnormal appendix as one with a MOD ≥7 mm and a maximal wall thickness ≥1.7 mm [35]. Secondary signs included hyperechogenic periappendiceal fat, fluid collection consistent with abscess, and local dilation and hypoperistalsis of bowel. For their final impression, radiologists were required to choose between four categories: (1) normal appendix, (2) appendix not visualized or partially visualized without secondary signs of appendicitis, (3) appendix not visualized or partially visualized with secondary signs of appendicitis, and (4) acute appendicitis. Categories 3 and 4 were considered positive for appendicitis. This template nearly eliminated nondiagnostic exams and improved diagnostic accuracy. Sensitivity improved from 67% to 92%. In other studies, the use of U/S templates has reduced use of CT, improved diagnostic accuracy, and reduced costs [36–38].

Rapidity of the test and repeatability are additional benefits of U/S. Increased sensitivity with increased duration of abdominal pain and repeated scans has been reported [39, 40]. U/S alone and in conjunction with algorithms that include U/S first have demonstrated lower costs and decreased use of CT [41–45]. The trend toward increased U/S use has not produced a concomitant increase in negative appendectomies, time to surgery, perforations, or missed appendicitis [4, 46–48].

Computed Tomography

CT findings of appendicitis are similar to those seen on U/S: appendiceal MOD >6 mm, increased wall thickness (target sign), wall hyperemia, periappendiceal mesenteric fat stranding, presence of an appendicolith, free fluid, and abscess [49]. Figure 5.2 demonstrates imaging by CT of confirmed appendicitis. Non-visualization of the appendix is possible on CT and argues against appendicitis with a very high (99%) negative predictive value [50]. The advantages of CT are its high sensitivity and specificity, operator independence, relatively quick acquisition time, widespread availability, and ability to identify alternate diagnoses.

CT has strong test characteristics in all populations, somewhat better than U/S, with a sensitivity of 0.90–0.95 and specificity of 0.92–0.95 (Table 5.1) [9, 13, 14]. Sensitivity and specificity improve slightly with intravenous contrast, but enteric contrast is generally unnecessary [51]. In children, however, several systematic reviews have shown that the sensitivity and specificity of CT are similar to U/S [9, 15]. CT's lower performance in children is due to relative lack of body fat, which makes distinguishing the appendix from surrounding structures more difficult [10, 52, 53]. In

Fig. 5.2 CT scan
demonstrates dilated
appendix (solid arrow)
with periappendiceal
mesenteric fat stranding
(hollow arrow)

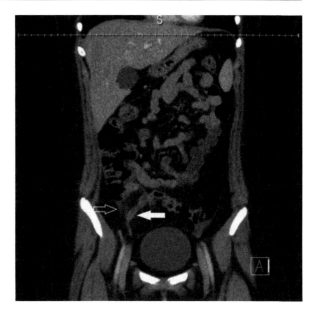

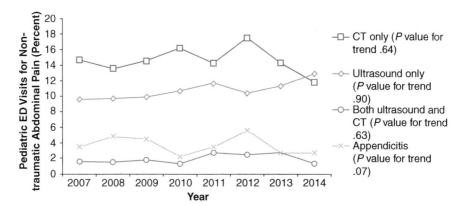

Fig. 5.3 Imaging trends in the United States for pediatric abdominal pain patients presenting to
the emergency department [55]

contrast to U/S, CT's high sensitivity and specificity remain consistent across institutions. In their meta-analysis of 9, 356 pediatric patients, Doria et al. reported little
variation between hospitals of institution-specific sensitivity and specificity [10].

CT is now ubiquitous in the United States, with more than 34 scanners per million
population as of 2007 [54]. Fourteen percent of children presenting to the emergency
department with non-traumatic abdominal pain undergo CT (Fig. 5.3) [55]. Being
faster than MRI, CT is useful for obtaining high-quality imaging in younger children,
who may not be able to remain still a prolonged time period. However, CT completion
may take significantly longer than U/S from time of order to performance [56]. CT

also identifies extra-appendiceal findings suggestive of other diagnoses more often than U/S [57, 58]. Because of these properties, CT may reduce the rate of negative appendectomies in children younger than 5 and girls older than 10 years of age [59].

Despite strong test characteristics, ease, and efficiency of performance, the ionizing radiation produced by CT raises concern. Focused exams and low-dose techniques, which have demonstrated equivalence to traditional techniques, have reduced radiation exposure but cannot eliminate it [60]. Children are particularly vulnerable to the effects of radiation, as their developing tissues are more sensitive and they have a longer remaining life span during which oncogenic effects may manifest [61]. Age at time of exposure impacts the risk of malignancy, with age inversely related to risk [62]. With growing recognition of the harms of healthcare-associated pediatric radiation exposure, limiting the utilization of CT is strongly recommended by national bodies such as the American College of Radiologists, the National Cancer Institute, the American Academy of Pediatrics, the American Pediatric Surgical Association, the Image Gently Alliance, and the Joint Commission [61, 63–66].

In the United States, individuals are exposed to approximately 3 mSv of background radiation per year. For reference, 1 mSv is equivalent to 1 mGy if the radiation type is gamma rays. An abdominal CT scan delivering 10 mSv is expected to cause cancer in the lifetime of 1 in 1000 male patients who are 10 years old at the time of imaging [67]. An estimated 4–9 million CT scans are performed annually on US children, 11% of which are obtained to evaluate for appendicitis [68, 69]. One year's worth of pediatric CTs is projected to cause 4870 cancers, but the true risk is unknown [70].

CT use in pediatric patients is associated with community, non-children's hospitals (NCH), older children, females, and patients with higher body mass index [71, 72]. Multiple studies have demonstrated that NCHs are more likely than children's hospitals (CH) to utilize CT to diagnose pediatric appendicitis [71–73]. The majority of pediatric patients with suspected appendicitis undergo CT, likely because 66–82% of these patients initially present to community and NCHs [74, 75]. Anderson et al. have also showed that the size-specific dose estimate and effective dose of radiation are significantly higher and have greater variance at NCHs that are not involved in a dose reduction program (Fig. 5.4) [76, 77].

CHs have led the effort to reduce CT utilization in children. As MRI has become increasingly available, it has begun to replace CT as a secondary modality after inconclusive U/S and is less commonly used as the primary study [72]. In addition to the radiation risk, CT use is not associated with better patient outcomes [78]. Other disadvantages of CT compared to U/S include cost and potential for allergic reaction or kidney injury from iodinated contrast agents. With radiation dose being cumulative, repeat CTs are not recommended.

Magnetic Resonance Imaging

The diagnostic features of appendicitis on MRI are similar to those previously mentioned. A study by Leeuwenburgh et al. described nine MRI features predictive of appendicitis: appendix diameter >7 mm, appendicolith, periappendiceal fat

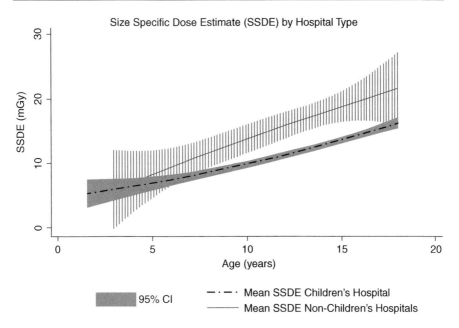

Fig. 5.4 Size-specific dose estimate by patient age at children's hospitals compared to non-children's hospitals [76]

infiltration, periappendiceal fluid, absence of gas in the appendix, appendiceal wall destruction, restricted diffusion of the appendiceal wall, and lumen or focal fluid collections [79]. Systematic reviews and meta-analyses have reported sensitivity from 0.96 to 0.99 and specificity ranging from 0.96 to 0.97 (Table 5.1) [9, 16–18]. In addition to strong test characteristics, MRI is also operator independent, provides alternative diagnoses as frequently as CT, and does not expose patients to ionizing radiation [80]. Figure 5.5 shows an MRI demonstrating appendicitis.

MRI does have several limitations, especially in the pediatric population. MRI may take longer to perform than either U/S or CT. The youngest children, those who cannot cooperate, or those with claustrophobia may require sedation to complete the exam. MRI is not as widely available as the other modalities and is more expensive as a stand-alone test than its comparators.

Traditional MRIs, with or without contrast, take longer to perform than U/S or CT. However, at centers where it is available, "fast" MRI has mitigated this problem. 3-T MRI produces a magnetic field twice as powerful as the more common 1.5T MRI, which typically decreases scanning time by half while retaining strong test characteristics [81]. In combination with 3-T MRI machines, parallel processing and newer body coils aid in reducing scan time, making it possible to scan children with free breathing, no IV contrast, and no sedation [82]. The benefit of gadolinium enhanced images has not been conclusively established [17, 83, 84].

Fig. 5.5 MRI
demonstrates dilated
appendix with
periappendiceal
enhancement consistent
with inflammation

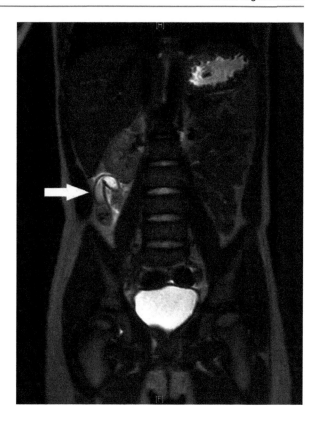

MRI is not as widely available as CT or U/S [54]. Hospital characteristics such as higher total expenditures and network affiliation are associated with its availability [85]. Even where available, MRI use has increased very slowly, comprising only 1–2% of all imaging for suspected appendicitis [47]. Otero et al., in a large retrospective study of trends and costs over time, found that while imaging costs of all studies increased slightly, it was at a much lower rate than overall hospital costs [47]. However, MRI only accounted for approximately 1% of imaging in that review. Heverhagen et al. reported that MRI is cost-effective as an isolated imaging modality because it decreases the rate of negative laparotomy, but their study did not compare MRI to U/S or CT [86]. Anderson et al. demonstrated a small, yet significant, increase in radiology costs with a large increase in MRI use (from 1% to 25%) in a single institution [46].

The utility of MRI as the first imaging test for appendicitis has not been established; nevertheless, it is a reliable alternative to CT when U/S is inconclusive. The slow transition from CT to MRI as the secondary imaging modality has not shown a change in outcomes. Several studies have reported no difference in time to antibiotic administration, time to surgery, negative appendectomy, perforation rate, or length of stay [46, 82, 87]. Future studies are necessary to evaluate the repercussions of this change in imaging strategy.

Discussion

Imaging for suspicion of pediatric appendicitis has become a common practice in the United States. As a result, tolerance for negative appendectomies and missed diagnoses has significantly decreased. Based on the available literature and current guidelines, U/S should be the first-line imaging modality in children with suspected appendicitis [88, 89]. MRI, where available, should be considered as a second-line exam in lieu of CT. CT may be beneficial when MRI cannot be performed, in older or obese children and in exigent circumstances. Imaging for suspected appendicitis is cost-effective for the reduction of negative appendectomies and decreased length of stay [90].

Imaging is rarely performed in isolation of history and physical and laboratory tests. The incorporation of commonly performed blood tests, such as a complete blood count, has demonstrated improved predictive value when used in conjunction with U/S [91]. The Alvarado Score, the Pediatric Appendicitis Score (PAS), the Appendicitis Inflammatory Response (AIR) Score, and similar tools have been used with great success to triage patients for imaging, to choose the imaging modality, or to support imaging results [43, 92–96]. Saucier et al. used the PAS to selectively image pediatric patients with U/S first, while Bachur et al. integrated the PAS with U/S results to determine next steps [43, 97]. Blitman et al. found a negative predictive value of 99.6% in patients with a low Alvarado Score and inconclusive U/S [92].

There is strong evidence that clinical guidelines or pathways for the diagnosis of appendicitis are efficient and cost-effective; they also reduce radiation exposure even if CT is included in the algorithm [40, 43, 46, 82, 98, 99, 100]. Published pathways are varied but generally include an U/S first protocol [101]. The LeBonheur pathway, as described by Saucier et al., had a diagnostic accuracy of 94% and was shown to be the 2nd most cost-effective strategy compared to U/S of all patients, clinical judgment alone, CT of all patients, overnight observation with surgical evaluation, and no imaging [102]. U/S of all patients was the most cost-effective; however, stratification by PAS had improved diagnostic accuracy with only a moderate increase in cost. U/S as the initial imaging modality with CT or MRI reserved for inconclusive U/S results increases overall diagnostic accuracy and decreases cost without sacrificing time to antibiotics or surgery [103, 104].

Continuing Controversies and Areas for Study

The evidence supports the use of U/S as the first diagnostic imaging test in children with suspected appendicitis. The utility of MRI first or MRI second has not been conclusively established, and more studies are needed to evaluate MRI alone or as part of an algorithm. Moreover, the role of CT, in light of radiation concerns, has not been fully determined. Several authors have suggested that MRI should replace CT as the secondary imaging modality after inconclusive U/S, but this practice has not been widely implemented, and the repercussions of such a shift have not been fully investigated. The Cochrane Collaboration is in the process of conducting a systematic review and meta-analysis of U/S and MRI for the diagnosis of acute appendicitis [105, 106]. They are also conducting a systematic review for evidence of the benefit of CT for acute appendicitis in adults.

Case Example Discussion

The case mentioned in the beginning of this chapter highlights the conundrums of imaging for suspected appendicitis in children. In this female patient with right lower quadrant pain, multiple diagnoses must be considered, including appendicitis, gynecologic pathologies such as ovarian torsion, or mesenteric adenitis. An ultrasound should be ordered for this patient. If the ultrasound is inconclusive, the emergency physician ought to consider the characteristics of their facility, transfer logistics, and patient/family preferences prior to ordering additional or repeat imaging.

In this case you recommended an U/S, which was obtained first. It demonstrated free pelvic fluid but was nondiagnostic. After you discussed the U/S results, the emergency physician ordered an MRI of the abdomen and pelvis on your recommendation, which showed a dilated appendix with periappendiceal inflammation and a normal right ovary. The patient was started on antibiotics, and an appendectomy was successfully performed several hours later.

Conclusion

Imaging for suspected pediatric appendicitis is an invaluable diagnostic tool, but modality selection can be controversial. First-line U/S is the evidence-based recommendation of the authors and the American College of Radiology [88]. Additional imaging is at the discretion of the provider, and multiple factors should be considered including availability of secondary modalities, exam and laboratory findings, surgeon assessment, patient characteristics, and patient/family preference.

Clinical Pearls

- Imaging is a valuable tool that has significantly improved our ability to correctly diagnose appendicitis and lower our negative appendectomy rate.
- U/S is a useful and safe first-line mode of imaging, but is operator dependent.
- MRI may provide a nonionizing radiation imaging option with a similar accuracy to CT scan.

References

1. Agency for Healthcare Research and Quality. HCUPnet: a tool for identifying, tracking, and analyzing national hospital statistics [Internet]. 2011. Available from: http://hcupnet.ahrq.gov/
2. Kaiser S, Mesas-Burgos C, Söderman E, Frenckner B. Appendicitis in children – impact of US and CT on the negative appendectomy rate. Eur J Pediatr Surg [Internet]. 2004;14(4):260–4. Available from: http://www.ncbi.nlm.nih.gov/pubmed/15343467

3. Puylaert JB. Acute appendicitis: US evaluation using graded compression. Radiology. 1986;158(2):355–60.
4. Bachur RG, Levy JA, Callahan MJ, Rangel SJ, Monuteaux MC. Effect of reduction in the use of computed tomography on clinical outcomes of appendicitis. JAMA Pediatr [Internet]. 2015;02115(8):1–6. Available from: http://archpedi.jamanetwork.com/article. aspx?doi=10.1001/jamapediatrics.2015.0479%5Cn; http://www.ncbi.nlm.nih.gov/ pubmed/26098076%5Cn; http://archpedi.jamanetwork.com/data/Journals/PEDS/0/ poi150021.pdf
5. Raja AS, Wright C, Sodickson AD, Zane RD, Schiff GD, Hanson R, et al. Negative appendectomy rate in the era of CT: an 18-year perspective. Radiology [Internet]. 2010;256(2):460–5. Available from: http://www.ncbi.nlm.nih.gov/pubmed/20529988
6. Kotagal M, Richards M, Flum D, Acierno S, Weinsheimer R, Goldin A. Use and accuracy of diagnostic imaging in the evaluation of pediatric appendicitis. J Pediatr Surg [Internet]. 2015;50(4):642–6. Available from: http://www.embase.com/search/results?subaction=viewr ecord&from=export&id=L603516778%5Cn, https://doi.org/10.1016/j. jpedsurg.2014.09.080%5Cn, http://elvis.ubvu.vu.nl:9003/vulink?sid=EMBASE&issn=1531 5037&id=doi:10.1016/j.jpedsurg.2014.09.080&atitle=Use+and+ac
7. Searle AR, Ismail KA, Macgregor D, Hutson JM. Changes in the length and diameter of the normal appendix throughout childhood. J Pediatr Surg [Internet] 2013;48(7):1535–1539. Available from: https://doi.org/10.1016/j.jpedsurg.2013.02.035
8. Goldin AB, Khanna P, Thapa M, McBroom JA, Garrison MM, Parisi MT. Revised ultrasound criteria for appendicitis in children improve diagnostic accuracy. Pediatr Radiol. 2011;41(8):993–9.
9. Zhang H, Liao M, Chen J, Zhu D, Byanju S. Ultrasound, computed tomography or magnetic resonance imaging – which is preferred for acute appendicitis in children? A meta-analysis. Pediatr Radiol [Internet]. 2017;47(2):186–96. Available from: https://doi.org/10.1007/ s00247-016-3727-3
10. Doria AS, Moineddin R, Kellenberger CJ, Epelman M, Beyene J, Schuh S, et al. US or CT for diagnosis of appendicitis in children and adults? A meta-analysis. Radiology. 2006;241(1):83–94.
11. Lowe LH, Penney MW, Stein SM, Heller RM, Neblett WW, Shyr Y, et al. Unenhanced limited CT of the abdomen in the diagnosis of appendicitis in children: comparison with sonography. Am J Roentgenol. 2001;176(1):31–5.
12. Matthew Fields J, Davis J, Alsup C, Bates A, Au A, Adhikari S, et al. Accuracy of point-of-care ultrasonography for diagnosing acute appendicitis: a systematic review and meta-analysis. Acad Emerg Med. 2017;24(9):1124–36.
13. Sivit CJ, Applegate KE, Stallion A, Dudgeon DL, Salvator A, Schluchter M, et al. Imaging evaluation of suspected appendicitis in a pediatric population. Am J Roentgenol [Internet]. 2000;175(4):977–80. Available from: http://www.ncbi.nlm.nih.gov/pubmed/11000147
14. Xiong B, Zhong B, Li Z, Zhou F, Hu R, Feng Z, et al. Diagnostic accuracy of noncontrast CT in detecting acute appendicitis: a meta-analysis of prospective studies. Am Surg. 2015;81(6):626–9.
15. Dahabrehm I, Adam G, Halladay C, Steele D, Daiello L, Weiland L, et al. Diagnosis of right lower quadrant pain and suspected acute appendicitis. Agency Healthc Res Qual [Internet]. 2015;(157). Available from: https://www.effectivehealthcare.ahrq.gov/ehc/prod-ucts/528/2158/appendicitis-report-151214.pdf
16. Repplinger MD, Levy JF, Peethumnongsin E, Gussick ME, Svenson JE, Golden SK, et al. Systematic review and meta-analysis of the accuracy of MRI to diagnose appendicitis in the general population. J Magn Reson Imaging. 2016;43(6):1346–54.
17. Moore MM, Kulaylat AN, Hollenbeak CS, Engbrecht BW, Dillman JR, Methratta ST. Magnetic resonance imaging in pediatric appendicitis: a systematic review. Pediatr Radiol [Internet]. 2016;46(6):928–39. Available from: https://doi.org/10.1007/ s00247-016-3557-3
18. Duke E, Kalb B, Arif-Tiwari H, Daye ZJ, Gilbertson-Dahdal D, Keim SM, et al. A systematic review and meta-analysis of diagnostic performance of MRI for evaluation of acute appendicitis. Am J Roentgenol. 2016;206(3):508–17.

19. Trout AT, Sanchez R, Ladino-Torres MF, Pai DR, Strouse PJ. A critical evaluation of US for the diagnosis of pediatric acute appendicitis in a real-life setting: how can we improve the diagnostic value of sonography? Pediatr Radiol [Internet]. 2012;42(7):813–23. Available from: http://www.ncbi.nlm.nih.gov/pubmed/22947273%5Cn; http://www.ncbi.nlm.nih.gov/pubmed/22402833

20. Wiersma F, Toorenvliet BR, Bloem JL, Allema JH, Holscher HC. US examination of the appendix in children with suspected appendicitis: the additional value of secondary signs. Eur Radiol. 2009;19(2):455–61.

21. Junewick J, Dombrowski K, Woolpert L, Vandop S, Schreiner M, Sutton P, et al. Rate of and factors affecting sonographic visualization of the appendix in asymptomatic children. Emerg Radiol. 2013;20(2):135–8.

22. Mittal MK, Dayan PS, Macias CG, Bachur RG, Bennett J, Dudley NC, et al. Performance of ultrasound in the diagnosis of appendicitis in children in a multicenter cohort. Acad Emerg Med. 2013;20(7):697–702.

23. Cohen B, Bowling J, Midulla P, Shlasko E, Lester N, Rosenberg H, et al. The non-diagnostic ultrasound in appendicitis: is a non-visualized appendix the same as a negative study? J Pediatr Surg [Internet]. 2015;50(6):923–7. Available from: http://linkinghub.elsevier.com/retrieve/pii/S0022346815001839

24. Nah SA, Ong SS, Lim WX, Amuddhu SK, Tang PH, Low Y. Clinical relevance of the nonvisualized appendix on ultrasonography of the abdomen in children. J Pediatr [Internet]. 2017;182:164–169.e1. Available from: https://doi.org/10.1016/j.jpeds.2016.11.062

25. Trout AT, Sanchez R, Ladino-torres MF. Reevaluating the sonographic criteria for acute appendicitis in children : Acad Radiol [Internet] 2012;19(11):1382–94. Available from: https://doi.org/10.1016/j.acra.2012.06.014

26. Kim SH, Choi YH, Kim WS, Cheon JE, Kim IO. Acute appendicitis in children: ultrasound and CT findings in negative appendectomy cases. Pediatr Radiol. 2014;44(10):1243–51.

27. Chang ST, Jeffrey RB, Olcott EW. Three-step sequential positioning algorithm during sonographic evaluation for appendicitis increases appendiceal visualization rate and reduces CT use. AJR Am J Roentgenol. 2014;203(5):1006–12.

28. Alter SM, Walsh B, Lenehan PJ, Shih RD. Ultrasound for diagnosis of appendicitis in a community hospital emergency department has a high rate of nondiagnostic studies. J Emerg Med [Internet]. 2017;52(6):833–8. Available from: https://doi.org/10.1016/j.jemermed.2017.01.003

29. Sivit CJ, Applegate KE, Berlin SC, Myers MT, Stallion A, Dudgeon DL, et al. Evaluation of suspected appendicitis in children and young adults: helical CT. Radiology. 2000;216(2):430–3.

30. Hörmann M, Scharitzer M, Stadler A, Pokieser P, Puig S, Helbich T. Ultrasound of the appendix in children: is the child too obese? Eur Radiol [Internet]. 2003;13(6):1428–31. Available from: http://www.ncbi.nlm.nih.gov/pubmed/12764662

31. Puig S, Staudenherz A, Felder-Puig R, Paya K. Imaging of appendicitis in children and adolescents: useful or useless? A comparison of imaging techniques and a critical review of the current literature. Semin Roentgenol. 2008;43:22–8.

32. Butler M, Servaes S, Srinivasan A, Edgar JC, Del Pozo G, Darge K. US depiction of the appendix: role of abdominal wall thickness and appendiceal location. Emerg Radiol. 2011;18(6):525–31.

33. Yiğiter M, Kantarci M, Yalçin O, Yalçin A, Salman AB. Does obesity limit the sonographic diagnosis of appendicitis in children? J Clin Ultrasound. 2011;39(4):187–90.

34. Gongidi P, Bellah RD. Ultrasound of the pediatric appendix. Pediatr Radiol. 2017;47(9):1091–100.

35. Nielsen JW, Boomer L, Kurtovic K, Lee E, Kupzyk K, Mallory R, et al. Reducing computed tomography scans for appendicitis by introduction of a standardized and validated ultrasonography report template. J Pediatr Surg [Internet]. 2015;50(1):144–8. Available from: http://www.ncbi.nlm.nih.gov/pubmed/25598112

36. Nordin AB, Sales S, Nielsen JW, Adler B, Bates DG, Kenney B. Standardized ultrasound templates for diagnosing appendicitis reduce annual imaging costs. J Surg Res [Internet]. 2018;221(614):77–83. Available from: https://doi.org/10.1016/j.jss.2017.07.002

37. Fallon SC, Orth RC, Guillerman RP, Munden MM, Zhang W, Elder SC, et al. Development and validation of an ultrasound scoring system for children with suspected acute appendicitis. Pediatr Radiol [Internet]. 2015. Available from: http://link.springer.com/10.1007/s00247-015-3443-4
38. Larson DB, Trout AT, Fierke SR, Towbin AJ. Improvement in diagnostic accuracy of ultrasound of the pediatric appendix through the use of equivocal interpretive categories. AJR Am J Roentgenol [Internet]. 2015;204(4):849–56. Available from: http://www.ncbi.nlm.nih.gov/pubmed/25794076
39. Bachur RG, Dayan PS, Bajaj L, MacIas CG, Mittal MK, Stevenson MD, et al. The effect of abdominal pain duration on the accuracy of diagnostic imaging for pediatric appendicitis. Ann Emerg Med [Internet]. 2012;60(5):582–590.e3. Available from: https://doi.org/10.1016/j.annemergmed.2012.05.034
40. Schuh S, Chan K, Langer JC, Kulik D, Preto-Zamperlini M, Aswad NA, et al. Properties of serial ultrasound clinical diagnostic pathway in suspected appendicitis and related computed tomography use. Acad Emerg Med. 2015;22:1–9.
41. Ramarajan N, Krishnamoorthi R, Barth R, Ghanouni P, Mueller C, Dannenburg B, et al. An interdisciplinary initiative to reduce radiation exposure: evaluation of appendicitis in a pediatric emergency department with clinical assessment supported by a staged ultrasound and computed tomography pathway. Acad Emerg Med. 2009;16(11):1258–65.
42. Krishnamoorthi R, Ramarajan N, Wang NE, Newman B, Rubesova E, Mueller CM, et al. Effectiveness of a staged US and CT protocol for the diagnosis of pediatric appendicitis: reducing radiation exposure in the age of ALARA. Radiology [Internet]. 2011;259(1):231–9. Available from: http://pubs.rsna.org/doi/10.1148/radiol.10100984
43. Saucier A, Huang EY, Emeremni CA, Pershad J. Prospective evaluation of a clinical pathway for suspected appendicitis. Pediatrics [Internet]. 2014;133(1):e88–95. Available from: http://www.ncbi.nlm.nih.gov/pubmed/24379237
44. Luo C-C, Chien W-K, Huang C-S, Lo H-C, Wu S-M, Huang H-C, et al. Trends in diagnostic approaches for pediatric appendicitis: nationwide population-based study. BMC Pediatr [Internet]. 2017;17(1):188. Available from: http://bmcpediatr.biomedcentral.com/articles/10.1186/s12887-017-0940-7
45. Kharbanda AB, Dudley NC, Bajaj L, Stevenson MD, Macias CG, Mittal MK, et al. Validation and refinement of a prediction rule to identify children at low risk for acute appendicitis. Arch Pediatr Adolesc Med [Internet]. 2012;166(8):738–44. Available from: http://www.pubmedcentral.nih.gov/articlerender.fcgi?artid=3790639&tool=pmcentrez&rendertype=abstract
46. Anderson K, Bartz-Kurycki M, Austin M, Kawaguchi A, John S, Kao L, et al. Approaching zero: implications of a computed tomography reduction program for pediatric appendicitis evaluation. J Pediatr Surg. 2017;52:1909–15.
47. Otero HJ, Crowder L. Imaging utilization for the diagnosis of appendicitis in stand-alone children's hospitals in the United States: trends and costs. J Am Coll Radiol [Internet]. 2017;1(6). Available from: https://doi.org/10.1016/j.jacr.2016.12.013
48. Lee J, Ko Y, Ahn S, Park JH, Kim HJ, Hwang SS, et al. Comparison of US and CT on the effect on negative appendectomy and appendiceal perforation in adolescents and adults: a post-hoc analysis using propensity-score methods. J Clin Ultrasound. 2016;44(7):401–10.
49. Choi D, Park H, Lee YR, Kook SH, Kim SK, Kwag HJ, et al. The most useful findings for diagnosing acute appendicitis on contrast-enhanced helical CT. Acta Radiol. 2003;44(6):574–82.
50. Garcia K, Hernanz-schulman M, Bennett DL, Morrow SE, Kan JH. Suspected appendicitis in children: diagnostic importance of normal abdominopelvic CT findings with nonvisualized appendix. Radiology. 2009;250(2):531–7.
51. Rentea RM, Peter SDS, Snyder CL. Pediatric appendicitis: state of the art review. Pediatr Surg Int. 2017;33(3):269–83.
52. Acheson J, Banerjee J. Management of suspected appendicitis in children. Arch Dis Child Educ Pract [Internet]. 2010;95(1):9–13. Available from: http://ep.bmj.com/cgi/doi/10.1136/adc.2009.168468
53. Friedland JA, Siegel MJ. CT appearance of acute appendicitis in childhood. Am J Roentgenol. 1997;168(2):439–42.

54. OECD. Number of magnetic resonance imaging (MRI) units and computed tomography (CT) scanners. Health (Irvine Calif) [Internet]. 2010;120:363–4. Available from: http://www.cdc. gov/nchs/data/hus/2010/120.pdf

55. Niles LM, Goyal MK, Badolato GM, Chamberlain JM, Cohen JS. US emergency department trends in imaging for pediatric nontraumatic abdominal pain. Pediatrics [Internet]. 2017;140(4):e20170615. Available from: http://pediatrics.aappublications.org/lookup/ doi/10.1542/peds.2017-0615%0A, http://www.ncbi.nlm.nih.gov/pubmed/28916590

56. Reich B, Zalut T, Weiner SG. An international evaluation of ultrasound vs. computed tomography in the diagnosis of appendicitis. Int J Emerg Med. 2011;4(1):1–7.

57. Halverson M, Delgado J, Mahboubi S. Extra-appendiceal findings in pediatric abdominal CT for suspected appendicitis. Pediatr Radiol. 2014;44(7):816–20.

58. Hernanz-Schulman M. CT and US in the diagnosis of appendicitis: an argument for CT. Radiology. 2010;255(1):3–7.

59. Bachur RG, Hennelly K, Callahan MJ, Chen C, Monuteaux MC. Diagnostic imaging and negative appendectomy rates in children: effects of age and gender. Pediatrics [Internet]. 2012;129(5):877–84. Available from: http://pediatrics.aappublications.org/cgi/doi/10.1542/ peds.2011-3375

60. Kim K, Kim YH, Kim SY, Kim S, Lee YJ, Kim KP, et al. Low-dose abdominal CT for evaluating suspected appendicitis. N Engl J Med [Internet]. 2012;366(17):1596–605. Available from: http://www.nejm.org/doi/abs/10.1056/NEJMoa1110734

61. Brody AS, Frush DP, Huda W, Brent RL. Radiation risk to children from computed tomography. Pediatrics. 2007;120(3):677–82.

62. Goske M, Applegate K, Frush D, Schulman MH, Morrison G. CT scans in childhood and risk of leukaemia and brain tumours. Lancet [Internet]. 2012;380(9855):1737–8. Available from: https://doi.org/10.1016/S0140-6736(12)61980-1

63. Cohen MD. ALARA, image gently and CT-induced cancer. Pediatr Radiol [Internet]. 2015;465–70. Available from: http://link.springer.com/10.1007/s00247-014-3198-3

64. Nosek AE, Hartin CW, Bass KD, Glick PL, Caty MG, Dayton MT, et al. Are facilities following best practices of pediatric abdominal CT scans? J Surg Res [Internet]. 2013;181(1):11–5. Available from: https://doi.org/10.1016/j.jss.2012.05.036

65. National Cancer Institute. Radiation risks and pediatric computed tomography – National Cancer Institute [Internet]. Society of pediatric radiology. 2012. Available from: http://www. cancer.gov/cancertopics/causes-prevention/risk/radiation/pediatric-ct-scans

66. American Academy of Pediatrics. AAP – No CT scans to evaluate abdominal pain Choosing Wisely [Internet]. Choosing Wisely. 2013. Available from: http://www.choosingwisely.org/ clinician-lists/american-academy-pediatrics-ct-scans-to-evaluate-abdominal-pain/

67. National Research Council. 2006. Health risks from exposure to low levels of ionizing radiation: BEIR VII Phase 2. Washington, DC: The National Academies Press. https://doi. org/10.17226/11340.

68. Brenner DJ, Elliston CD, Hall EJ, Berdon WE. Estimated risks of radiation-induced fatal cancer from pediatric CT. AJR. 2001;176(2):289–96.

69. Brenner DJ, Hall EJ. Computed tomography – an increasing source of radiation exposure. N Engl J Med. 2007;357(22):2277–84.

70. Miglioretti DL, Johnson E, Williams A, Greenlee RT, Weinmann S, Solberg LI, et al. The use of computed tomography in pediatrics and the associated radiation exposure and estimated cancer risk. JAMA Pediatr [Internet]. 2013;167(8):700–7. Available from: http://www.ncbi. nlm.nih.gov/pubmed/23754213

71. Glass CC, Saito JM, Sidhwa F, Cameron DB, Feng C, Karki M, et al. Diagnostic imaging practices for children with suspected appendicitis evaluated at de fi nitive care hospitals and their associated referral centers. J Pediatr Surg [Internet]. 2016;51(6):912–6. Available from: https://doi.org/10.1016/j.jpedsurg.2016.02.055

72. Anderson K, Bartz-Kurycki M, Austin M, Kawaguchi A, Kao LS, Lally KP, et al. Hospital type predicts computed tomography use for pediatric appendicitis. J Pediatr Surg. 2018;54(4):723–7.

73. Tinsley Anderson K, Putnam LR, Caldwell KM, Diffley MB, Hildebrandt AA, Covey SE, et al. Imaging gently? Higher rates of computed tomography imaging for pediatric appendicitis in non–children's hospitals. Surgery [Internet]. 2016;161(5):1326–33. Available from: https://doi.org/10.1016/j.surg.2016.09.042

74. Tian Y, Heiss KF, Wulkan ML, Raval MV. Assessment of variation in care and outcomes for pediatric appendicitis at children's and non-children's hospitals. J Pediatr Surg [Internet]. 2015;50(11):1885–92. Available from: http://linkinghub.elsevier.com/retrieve/pii/S0022346815003905

75. Rice-Townsend S, Barnes JN, Hall M, Baxter JL, Rangel SJ. Variation in practice and resource utilization associated with the diagnosis and management of appendicitis at freestanding children's hospitals: implications for value-based comparative analysis. Ann Surg. 2014;6(259):1228–34. Available from: http://www.ncbi.nlm.nih.gov/pubmed/24096770

76. Anderson KT, Greenfield S, Putnam LR, Hamilton E, Kawaguchi A, Austin MT, et al. Don't forget the dose: improving computed tomography dosing for pediatric appendicitis. J Pediatr Surg. 2016;51:1944–8.

77. Kim ME, Orth RC, Fallon SC, Lopez ME, Brandt ML, Zhang W, et al. Performance of CT examinations in children with suspected acute appendicitis in the community setting: a need for more education. Am J Roentgenol [Internet]. 2015;204(4):857–60. Available from: http://www.ajronline.org/doi/10.2214/AJR.14.12750

78. Miano D, Silvis R, Popp J, Culbertson M, Campbell B, Smith S. Abdominal CT does not improve outcome for children with suspected acute appendicitis. West J Emerg Med. 2015;16(7):974–82.

79. Leeuwenburgh MMN, Jensch S, Gratama JWC, Spilt A, Wiarda BM, Van Es HW, et al. MRI features associated with acute appendicitis. Eur Radiol. 2014;24(1):214–22.

80. Dillman JR, Gadepalli S, Sroufe NS, Davenport MS, Smith EA, Chong ST, et al. Equivocal pediatric appendicitis: unenhanced MR imaging protocol for nonsedated children – a clinical effectiveness study. Radiology [Internet]. 2016;279(1):216–25. Available from: http://pubs.rsna.org/doi/10.1148/radiol.2015150941

81. Johnson AK, Filippi CG, Andrews T, Higgins T, Tam J, Keating D, et al. Ultrafast 3-T MRI in the evaluation of children with acute lower abdominal pain for the detection of appendicitis. Am J Roentgenol. 2012;198(6):1424–30.

82. Kulaylat AN, Moore MM, Engbrecht BW, Brian JM, Khaku A, Hollenbeak CS, et al. An implemented MRI program to eliminate radiation from the evaluation of pediatric appendicitis. J Pediatr Surg. 2015;50(8):1359–63.

83. Orth RC, Guillerman RP, Zhang W, Masand P, Iii GSB. Prospective comparison of MR imaging and US for the diagnosis of pediatric appendicitis. Radiology. 2014;272(1):233–40. Available from: http://pubs.rsna.org/doi/full/10.1148/radiol.14132206

84. Rosines LA, Chow DS, Lampl BS, Chen S, Gordon S, Mui LW, et al. Value of gadolinium-enhanced MRI in detection of acute appendicitis in children and adolescents. Am J Roentgenol [Internet]. 2014;203(5):W543–8. Available from: http://www.ajronline.org/doi/abs/10.2214/AJR.13.12093

85. Khaliq AA, Deyo D, Duszak R. The impact of hospital characteristics on the availability of radiology services at critical access hospitals. J Am Coll Radiol [Internet]. 2015;12(12):1351–6. Available from: https://doi.org/10.1016/j.jacr.2015.09.008

86. Heverhagen JT, Pfestroff K, Heverhagen AE, Klose KJ, Kessler K, Sitter H. Diagnostic accuracy of magnetic resonance imaging: a prospective evaluation of patients with suspected appendicitis (Diamond). J Magn Reson Imaging. 2012;35(3):617–23.

87. Aspelund G, Fingeret A, Gross E, Kessler D, Keung C, Thirumoorthi A, et al. Ultrasonography/MRI versus CT for diagnosing appendicitis. Pediatrics [Internet]. 2014;133(4):586–93. Available from: http://www.ncbi.nlm.nih.gov/pubmed/24590746

88. Zelop CM, Javitt MC, Glanc P, Dubinsky T, Harisinghani MG, Harris RD, et al. ACR Appropriateness Criteria® growth disturbances – risk of intrauterine growth restriction. Ultrasound Q. 2013;29(3):147–51.

89. Rosen MP, Ding A, Blake MA, Baker ME, Cash BD, Fidler JL, et al. ACR appropriateness Criteria® right lower quadrant painsuspected appendicitis. J Am Coll Radiol [Internet]. 2011;8(11):749–55. Available from: https://doi.org/10.1016/j.jacr.2011.07.010

90. Lahaye MJ, Lambregts DMJ, Mutsaers E, Essers BAB, Breukink S, Cappendijk VC, et al. Mandatory imaging cuts costs and reduces the rate of unnecessary surgeries in the diagnostic work-up of patients suspected of having appendicitis. Eur Radiol [Internet]. 2015;25(5):1464–70. Available from: http://link.springer.com/10.1007/s00330-014-3531-0

91. Anandalwar SP, Callahan MJ, Bachur RG, Feng C, Sidhwa F, Karki M, et al. Use of white blood cell count and polymorphonuclear leukocyte differential to improve the predictive value of ultrasound for suspected appendicitis in children. J Am Coll Surg [Internet]. 2015;220(6):1010–7. Available from: http://linkinghub.elsevier.com/retrieve/pii/S1072751515000940

92. Blitman NM, Anwar M, Brady KB, Taragin BH, Freeman K. Value of focused appendicitis ultrasound and alvarado score in predicting appendicitis in children: can we reduce the use of CT? Am J Roentgenol [Internet]. 2015;204(6):W707–12. Available from: http://www.ajronline.org/doi/10.2214/AJR.14.13212

93. Ohle R, O'Reilly F, O'Brien KK, Fahey T, Dimitrov BD. The Alvarado score for predicting acute appendicitis: a systematic review. BMC Med [Internet]. 2011;9(1):139. Available from: http://bmcmedicine.biomedcentral.com/articles/10.1186/1741-7015-9-139

94. Schneider C, Kharbanda A, Bachur R. Evaluating appendicitis scoring systems using a prospective pediatric cohort. Ann Emerg Med. 2007;49(6):778–84.

95. Samuel M. Pediatric appendicitis score. J Pediatr Surg. 2002;37(6):877–81.

96. Toprak H, Kilincaslan H, Ahmad IC, Yildiz S, Bilgin M, Sharifov R, et al. Integration of ultrasound findings with Alvarado score in children with suspected appendicitis. Pediatr Int. 2014;56(1):95–9.

97. Bachur RG, Callahan MJ, Monuteaux MC, Rangel SJ. Integration of ultrasound findings and a clinical score in the diagnostic evaluation of pediatric appendicitis. J Pediatr. 2015;166(5):1134–9.

98. Wagenaar AE, Tashiro J, Wang B, Curbelo M, Mendelson KL, Perez EA, et al. Protocol for suspected pediatric appendicitis limits computed tomography utilization. J Surg Res [Internet]. 2015;199(1):153–8. Available from: https://doi.org/10.1016/j.jss.2015.04.028

99. Woolf S, Schünemann HJ, Eccles MP, Grimshaw JM, Shekelle P. Developing clinical practice guidelines: types of evidence and outcomes; values and economics, synthesis, grading, and presentation and deriving recommendations. Implement Sci [Internet]. 2012;7(1):61. Available from: http://implementationscience.biomedcentral.com/articles/10.1186/1748-5908-7-61

100. Glass CC, Rangel SJ. Overview and diagnosis of acute appendicitis in children. Semin Pediatr Surg [Internet]. 2016;25(4):198–203. Available from: https://doi.org/10.1053/j.sempedsurg.2016.05.001

101. Russell WS, Schuh AM, Hill JG, Hebra A, Cina RA, Smith CD, et al. Clinical practice guidelines for pediatric appendicitis evaluation can decrease computed tomography utilization while maintaining diagnostic accuracy. Pediatr Emerg Care [Internet]. 2013;29(5):568–73. Available from: http://eutils.ncbi.nlm.nih.gov/entrez/eutils/elink.fcgi?dbfrom=pubmed&id=23611916&retmode=ref&cmd=prlinks

102. Taylor GA, Anderson KT, Greenfield S, Putnam LR, Hamilton E, Kawaguchi A, et al. Cost-effectiveness of diagnostic approaches to suspected appendicitis in children. J Pediatr Surg [Internet]. 2015;220(4):153–8. Available from: http://linkinghub.elsevier.com/retrieve/pii/S1072751514019115

103. Rosendahl K, Aukland SM, Fosse K. Imaging strategies in children with suspected appendicitis. Eur Radiol Suppl [Internet]. 2004;14(4):L138–45. Available from: http://link.springer.com/10.1007/s00330-003-2077-3

104. Imler D, Keller C, Sivasankar S, Wang NE, Vasanawala S, Bruzoni M, et al. MRI vs. Ultrasound as the initial imaging modality for pediatric and young adult patients with suspected appendicitis. Acad Emerg Med. 2017; Epub ahead (accepted author manuscript). https://doi.org/10.1111/acem.13180
105. Wild J, Abdul N, Ritchie J, Bo R, Freels S, Nelson R. Ultrasonography for diagnosis of acute appendicitis (Protocol). Cochrane Database Syst Rev 2013;(2).
106. D'Souza, et al. Cochrane Database of Systematic Reviews Magnetic resonance imaging (MRI) for diagnosis of acute appendicitis (Protocol) Magnetic resonance imaging (MRI) for diagnosis of acute appendicitis (Protocol). Cochrane Database Syst Rev Art [Internet]. 2016;(1). Available from: www.cochranelibrary.com

Selection and Timing of Antibiotics for the Management of Appendicitis

6

Christopher Gayer and Michelle V. L. Nguyen

Case Example

A 12-year-old girl presents to the emergency department with 2 days of abdominal pain that began centrally and has migrated to the right lower quadrant. Her mother reports a fever to 38 °C and multiple episodes of vomiting and diarrhea. On physical exam, the patient has focal peritonitis in the right lower quadrant. White blood cell count is 18,000 /uL, and C-reactive protein is 1.8 mg/L. Abdominal ultrasound demonstrates a 9 mm non-compressible, blind-ended tubular structure in the right lower quadrant and a moderate amount of free fluid in the pelvis, consistent with perforated appendicitis. Which antibiotics should be started, and for how long should they be continued?

Introduction

Appendicitis is one of the most common diseases that general surgeons manage. While antibiotic use is widely accepted and is considered current standard of care, there is little consensus regarding which class, route of administration, or duration of antibiotics is best. Furthermore, it is not clear if these choices actually work to resolve the ongoing intra-abdominal infection or reduce post-treatment complications as they are meant to. Many institutions have protocols directing a change in the antibiotic regimen depending on whether the patient's disease is complicated or uncomplicated. Simple or uncomplicated appendicitis typically refers to pathology limited to appendiceal inflammation, while complicated appendicitis generally

C. Gayer (✉) · M. V. L. Nguyen
Department of Surgery, Division of Pediatric Surgery, Keck School of Medicine of University of Southern California, Los Angeles, CA, USA

Children's Hospital of Los Angeles, Los Angeles, CA, USA
e-mail: cgayer@chla.usc.edu; micnguyen@chla.usc.edu

© Springer Nature Switzerland AG 2019
C. J. Hunter (ed.), *Controversies in Pediatric Appendicitis*,
https://doi.org/10.1007/978-3-030-15006-8_6

involves appendiceal perforation and/or intra-abdominal abscess formation. However, between these extremes is a spectrum of disease involving other features like gangrene, purulence, and presence of an obstructing appendiceal fecalith or appendicolith. Different studies often distinguish uncomplicated from complicated appendicitis at conflicting points along this spectrum, and sometimes also consider other factors, like delayed return of bowel function or requirement of intensive care, to be complicated. Because the label guides the antibiotic management in most institutions, the lack of universally agreed-upon criteria for complicated appendicitis makes reconciling individual studies and recommendations difficult. The details of antibiotic use in the treatment of appendicitis are not standardized. Herein we discuss the literature supporting common practices.

Current guidelines from multiple experts are similar but still ultimately conflicting. The Infectious Disease Society of America states that the routine use of broad-spectrum antibiotics is unnecessary if there is a high likelihood that the appendicitis is uncomplicated [1]. A recent Cochrane review also recommends narrow-spectrum antibiotics, suggesting that a first-generation cephalosporin with metronidazole or a second-generation cephalosporin alone is sufficient [2]. The Surgical Infection Society (SIS)'s 2017 guidelines on the management of intra-abdominal infection (not specific to appendicitis) specify using cefotaxime, ciprofloxacin plus metronidazole, or ertapenem for community-acquired infection due to a pathogen determined to be at low risk for antibiotic resistance. Recommendations are piperacillin-tazobactam, imipenem-cilastatin, or meropenem for community-acquired infection due to a pathogen at high risk for antibiotic resistance or hospital-acquired infection in children. Interestingly, by those authors' own admission, the definition of high and low risk of antibiotic resistance is vaguely defined and in practice would depend on specific antibiotic resistant patterns at a given institution. These same guidelines suggest a maximum of 5 days for children with adequate source control, but 7 days of intravenous antibiotics for the specific scenario of perforated appendicitis with intra-abdominal abscess [3]. However, the SIS's Study to Optimize Peritoneal Infection Therapy (STOP-IT) from the same year found that continuing antibiotics beyond 4 days made no difference in rates of surgical site infection, intra-abdominal infection, or death at 30 days after source control [4]. This study involved all causes of intra-abdominal infection, although about 10% of the patients included in the trial had appendicitis. Despite these findings, common practice in many institutions is to start broad-spectrum antibiotics, such as piperacillin-tazobactam, immediately at diagnosis, and then make adjustments based on the severity of infection observed at surgery. For uncomplicated appendicitis, the 2017 Pediatric Infectious Disease Journal recommends switching to ampicillin and gentamicin plus metronidazole or clindamycin, or ceftriaxone plus metronidazole until the patient tolerates oral antibiotics, followed by early discharge home on oral amoxicillin-clavulanate. For complicated appendicitis, the same journal recommends continuing piperacillin-tazobactam until the patient tolerates oral antibiotics [5]. At this author's home institution, a pediatric hospital, patients receive broad-spectrum antibiotics upon diagnosis. During appendectomy, the disease is categorized as acute (limited to peri-appendiceal inflammation without gross contamination of the peritoneal cavity), suppurative (contamination of the perito-neal cavity), gangrenous (appendiceal wall necrosis), or gross perforation. These categories are very similar, but not identical, to the American Association of Surgery for Trauma (AAST)'s severity grades for appendicitis, which Hernandez et al. vali-dated and found that increasing grade correlates with increasing complication sever-ity in children [6]. Piperacillin-tazobactam is discontinued for appendectomy demonstrating acute disease or continued for increasing durations correlating to the severity of disease and guided by laboratory data, regardless of oral intake.

One of the main controversies in appendicitis treatment protocols is the adequacy of narrow-spectrum antibiotics versus the necessity of broad-spectrum antibiotics. General principles for antibiotic use allow initial narrow-spectrum antibiotics if there is a historically likely causative bacteria with known susceptibilities. If the offending pathogen is unknown or the infection is severe, treatment begins with broad-spectrum antibiotics and is narrowed based on later culture results. However, cultures are not routinely performed for appendicitis. Furthermore, causative bacte-ria may be quite similar in the vast majority of cases. In a South Korean study of appendicitis, Song et al. found that 64.6% of the bacteria isolated from appendiceal lumens and intra-abdominal abscesses grew *E. coli* susceptible to most cephalospo-rins, ciprofloxacin, and broad-spectrum penicillins. Only 16.4% of isolated bacteria were *P. aeruginosa* resistant to cefotaxime and broad-spectrum penicillins, and these were associated with increased risk of superficial surgical site infections [7]. A worldwide study by Coccolini et al. corroborated that most bacteria isolated from appendicitis patients are gram-negative, specifically *E. coli*. Gram-positive bacteria were less prevalent, the most common being *Streptococcus*. Only 6.3% of gram-negative and 0.1% of gram-positive bacteria demonstrated notable resistance to narrow-spectrum antibiotics [8]. Taken together, these studies suggest that the caus-ative bacteria are often similar, and antibiotic resistance requiring broad-spectrum antibiotics is less common in patients with appendicitis.

In addition to resolving the primary appendiceal infection, antibiotics are most often used to reduce or prevent post-treatment complications, i.e. surgical site infec-tions and intra-abdominal abscesses. For uncomplicated appendicitis, Cameron et al. compared three antibiotic regimens: cefoxitin, ceftriaxone plus metronidazole, or piperacillin-tazobactam. They found no difference in incisional or organ-space surgical site infections, returns to the hospital, readmissions, or cost within 30 days of operation [2]. It seems reasonable to assume that complicated appendicitis – involving perforation and gross intra-abdominal contamination seen at the time of operation – would be more likely to result in post-treatment complications and therefore benefit from longer and broader-spectrum antibiotic treatment. Upon investigating this idea, however, Kronman et al. found that with regard to 30-day hospital readmission or requirement of additional abdominal procedures, broad-spectrum antibiotics (i.e., piperacillin-tazobactam, ticarcillin-clavulanate, ceftazi-dime, cefepime, or carbapenem in this study) offered no advantage over narrower-spectrum antibiotics (not specifically named) in post-appendectomy patients with uncomplicated or complicated appendicitis. Unlike most other studies, this one expanded its definition of "complicated appendicitis" to include a hospital stay greater than 3 days, requirement for central venous access, major or severe illness, or admission to an intensive care unit [9]. Another source of controversy that exists around antibiotic selection is the addition of an agent specifically targeting anaerobes. Shang et al. compared outcomes of perforated appendicitis treated with broad-spectrum antibiotics with and without the addition of metronidazole. This study found that metronidazole made no difference in the rate surgical wound infection, intra-abdominal abscess, or 30-day readmission when compared to broad-spectrum antibiotics alone. Additional outcomes that were unchanged by metronidazole included duration of intravenous antibiotics, hospital length of stay, and inflammatory markers on post-operative day 5 [10]. Taken together, these data suggest that narrow-spectrum antibiotics without anaerobic coverage are an adequate choice in the treatment of both uncomplicated and complicated appendicitis (Table 6.1). Regardless, it is difficult to overcome the intuition that more severe infections warrant broader-spectrum antibiotics. This author's home institution is a tertiary pediatric referral center that cares for a disproportionately higher percentage of complicated appendicitis. Current protocol directs all patients, except those with the mildest category of disease, to receive broad-spectrum antibiotics for at least 12 hours post-operatively.

Aside from the spectrum of coverage, the other main variable in an antibiotic regimen is the duration of treatment. As previously mentioned, the SIS suggests giving antibiotics for 4–5 days in a patient with source control and up to 7 days in a patient without source control [3, 4]. However, these recommendations are for general intra-abdominal infections. To determine the necessary antibiotic duration

Table 6.1 Summary of findings regarding antibiotic selection

First author, year	Treatment groups	Demographic, disease severity	Primary outcomes	Conclusion
Cameron D, 2017	Pip-tazo vs cefoxitin vs CTX + metronidazole	Pediatric, uncomplicated	30-day SSI (superficial, deep, organ space), returns to ED, hospital readmission	Extended spectrum not associated with decreased outcomes
Kronman M, 2016	Pip-tazo vs ticarcillin-clavulanate vs ceftazidime vs cefepime vs carbapenem	Pediatric, complicated and uncomplicated	30-day readmission for SSI or additional abdominal procedures	Extended spectrum offers no advantage
Shang Q, 2017	Broad-spectrum alone vs broad-spectrum + metronidazole	Pediatric, perforated	Postoperative antibiotic duration, POD5 WBC/CRP, LOS, intra-abdominal abscess, wound infection	Metronidazole has no beneficial clinical effects

Pip-tazo piperacillin-tazobactam, *CTX* ceftriaxone, *SSI* surgical site infection, *ED* emergency department, *POD* postoperative day, *WBC* white blood cell count, *CRP* C-reactive protein, *LOS* length of stay

Table 6.2 Summary of findings regarding antibiotic duration

First author, year	Treatment groups	Demographic, disease severity	Primary outcomes	Conclusion
Sawyer R, 2015	Abx for 4 ± 1 day vs abx until 2 days after resolution of fever, leukocytosis, and ileus (maximum 10 days)	Adult, not specific to appendicitis	30-day SSI, recurrent intra-abdominal infection, death	No significant difference
van Rossem C, 2016	3 vs 5 days of postoperative abx	Pediatric and adult, complicated	SSI, intra-abdominal abscess, postoperative ileus	5 days not associated with reduced infectious complications
Kim D, 2015	Postoperative abx vs no postoperative abx	Adult, gangrenous and perforated	Wound complications, LOS, hospital readmission	Postoperative abx associated with increased LOS but not decreased wound complications

Abx antibiotics

specifically for pediatric appendicitis, van Rossem et al. compared the rate of infectious complications including surgical site infection, intra-abdominal abscess, and post-operative ileus in children with complicated appendicitis who received 3 versus 5 days of postoperative antibiotics, whether entirely intravenous or combined intravenous-oral. Their definition of "complicated" appendicitis included patients whose surgeons prescribed post-operative antibiotics for greater than 24 hours for any reason, which suggests a subset of patients thought to have more severe infection than average. They found no difference in infectious complications in groups receiving 3 days of postoperative antibiotics compared to 5 [11]. Taken together, these studies suggest that following appendectomy, antibiotics should not be continued after postoperative day 5 and may be stopped as early as postoperative day 3 (Table 6.2).

Other questions related to antibiotic spectrum and duration include whether antibiotics are necessary after discharge from the hospital, and if the oral or intravenous route is superior. Generally, oral antibiotics are narrower spectrum and are given after control of the infectious source. In uncomplicated appendicitis, this typically means immediately post-operatively, after appendectomy. Patients with complicated appendicitis may receive oral home antibiotics or may require intravenous home antibiotics (the latter is especially common if source control was not possible due to degree of perforation). In a study comparing rates of complications after discharge home on oral versus intravenous antibiotics for perforated appendicitis in post-appendectomy patients, Rangel et al. found that treatment failure (defined as organ-space infection requiring percutaneous or operative drainage) and all-cause hospital revisits or admissions (e.g., wound complications, bowel obstruction, intravenous catheter complications) were more frequent in patients receiving intravenous home antibiotics [12]. This may have resulted from selection bias, since the patients determined likely to benefit from intravenous home antibiotics are usually those with more severe infections as determined by clinical criteria, such as intra-operative findings, persistent fever, or leukocytosis during post-operative monitoring. Although those authors minimize this disease severity-based confounding by matching patients with similar severity-associated characteristics, they acknowledge the potential for residual effects. Importantly, the study did not show that intravenous home antibiotics reduced the rate of post-operative complications in perforated appendicitis, which suggests that even in very severe disease, systemic treatment with broad-spectrum antibiotics may not make a difference in complication rate.

While predetermined, evidence-based protocols for antibiotic selection and timing are useful starting points, an often-employed adjunct is to allow patients' clinical features to guide development of individualized antibiotic regimens. For example, a patient with post-operative fever and/or leukocytosis may be deemed still acutely ill and thus receive a longer antibiotic duration. Evidence supporting use of persistently elevated serum inflammatory markers such as white blood cell count (WBC) and the acute phase reactant C-reactive protein (CRP) are conflicting. The previously mentioned STOP-IT trial suggests that a prolonged systemic inflammatory response syndrome after 4 days may be reflective of simply ongoing immune activity and not necessarily indicative of ongoing bacterial presence [4]. However, other studies, including work from Assarsson et al., found a significant correlation between improvement in WBC and CRP within 24 hours of starting antibiotics and improvement of clinical disease. The correlation between resolution of fever and resolution of disease was not significant ($p = 0.06$) [13]. Procalcitonin (PCT) is another acute phase reactant that has shown promise as a marker of specifically bacteria-induced inflammation and systemic shock. There is especially a fast-growing support for use of elevated serum PCT levels as an indicator to continue antibiotics in lower respiratory bacterial infections like bronchitis and pneumonia, while de-escalating or stopping antibiotics based on decreasing PCT levels improves respiratory and ICU outcomes [14]. Theoretically, PCT levels could also aid in tailoring individualized antibiotic regimens for intra-abdominal bacterial infections, but existing data in this context is new and therefore meager. Assarsson et al. compared PCT levels in appendicitis patients who were clinically responding to antibiotics versus PCT levels in patients who were deemed antibiotic non-responders, but they found no difference in these groups, concluding that PCT is not a useful predictor of antibiotic response [13]. Similarly, Slieker et al. queried whether elevated serum PCT levels might help identify patients with peritonitis who are likely to develop postoperative complications but found that PCT levels did not correlate to differences in required antibiotic duration, hospital length of stay, rate of postoperative complications, or death [14]. However, conclusions about PCT levels in the specific context of intra-abdominal infections and appendicitis are at best undefined, and this topic may be of interest for future study. Meanwhile, despite a lack of definitive supporting evidence, post-operative fever, leukocytosis, and elevated CRP remain widely trusted indicators of ongoing infection. If the patient in the case study were a current patient at this author's home institution and had a WBC greater than 15 on post-operative day 3, she would receive further intravenous antibiotics.

If she were still febrile on the evening of post-operative day 2, her WBC would not be checked until she had been afebrile for 24 hours.

Because appendicitis is an inflammatory condition with associated infection, antibiotics have long been commonplace in the care of patients with this disease, prompting continued debate over the details. These details include the previously discussed broadness of coverage, route of administration, and duration. However, with current efforts to decrease bacterial development of antibiotic resistance by reducing antibiotic usage, it is interesting to consider whether the diagnosis of appendicitis really warrants antibiotic treatment at all. In a randomized controlled trial, Park et al. treated computed tomography-verified, uncomplicated appendicitis in adults with either intravenous second-generation cephalosporin plus metronidazole or supportive care and intravenous vitamins for 4 days. This study found that between treatment groups, there was no difference in requirement of drainage, surgery, or further antibiotics within 1 month. Additionally, patients in the supportive care group had decreased length of hospital stay and overall cost [15]. However, in 2017, a meta-analysis involving pediatric patients with uncomplicated appendicitis found that non-operative management with antibiotics resulted in increased hospital readmissions, concluding that appendectomy at the time of index admission is still the treatment of choice in this population [16]. Interestingly, a study investigating the necessity of post-operative antibiotics for complicated appendicitis in adults by Kim et al. also found no difference in hospital readmission or superficial or deep surgical site infection. The finding of decreased length of hospital stay for patients not receiving antibiotics continued to hold true for the adult complicated appendicitis cohort [17]. Similar studies are currently ongoing at major academic centers in the United States.

Conclusions

Although appendicitis is considered a classic surgical diagnosis, and the frequency at which surgeons encounter it makes its management one of the foremost items in training surgeons' repertoires, there still exists wide, often institution-specific variation in its treatment. Regardless of the antibiotic regimen or protocol used, the guiding principle remains to reduce broadness of coverage, invasiveness of administration, and duration as much as possible while still minimizing these patients' postoperative morbidity. Despite sometimes conflicting or unclear data, our best recommendation based on the available literature is to treat all appendicitis, regardless of severity, with narrower-spectrum antibiotics for 3 days postoperatively, unless persistently elevated WBC and/or CRP suggest the patient may benefit from extending the treatment for a maximum of 5 total days.

Clinical Pearls

- Initiate antibiotics in a timely fashion following diagnosis.
- Reduce the broadness and duration of antibiotics as much as possible.
- WBC and/or CRP level may aid in deciding when to discontinue antibiotics.

References

1. Mueck K, Putnam L, Anderson K, Lally K, Tsao K, Kao L. Does compliance with antibiotic prophylaxis in pediatric simple appendicitis matter? J Surg Res. 2017;216:1–8.
2. Cameron D, Melvin P, Graham D, Glass C, Serres S, Kronman M, Saito J, Rangel S. Extended versus narrow-spectrum antibiotics in the management of uncomplicated appendicitis in children. Ann Surg. 2017;268(1):186–92.
3. Mazuski J, Tessier J, May A, et al. The surgical infection society revised guidelines on the management of intra-abdominal infection. Surg Infect. 2017;18:1–76.
4. Sawyer R, Claridge J, Nathens A, et al. Trial of short-course antimicrobial therapy for intraabdominal infection. N Engl J Med. 2015;372:1996–2005.
5. Willis Z, Duggan E, Gillon J, Blakely M, Di Pentima M. Improvements in antimicrobial prescribing and outcomes in pediatric complicated appendicitis. Pediatr Infect Dis J. 2018;37:429–35.
6. Hernandez M, Polites S, Aho J, Haddad N, Kong V, Saleem H, Bruce J, Laing G, Clarke D, Zielinski M. Measuring anatomic severity in pediatric appendicitis: validation of the American Association for the Surgery of Trauma appendicitis severity grade. J Pediatr. 2018;192:229–33.
7. Song D, Park B, Suh S, et al. Bacterial culture and antibiotic susceptibility in patients with acute appendicitis. Int J Color Dis. 2018;33:441–7.
8. Coccolini F, D'Amico G, Sartelli M, Catena F, Montori G, Ceresoli M, Manfredi R, Di Saverio S, Ansaloni L. Antibiotic resistance evaluation and clinical analysis of acute appendicitis; report of 1431 consecutive worldwide patients: a cohort study. Int J Surg. 2016;26:6–11.
9. Kronman M, Oron A, Ross R, Hersh A, Newland J, Goldin A, Rangel S, Weissman S, Zerr D, Gerber J. Extended- versus narrower-spectrum antibiotics for appendicitis. Pediatrics. 2016;138:e20154547.
10. Shang Q, Geng Q, Zhang X, Guo C. The efficacy of combined therapy with metronidazole and broad-spectrum antibiotics on postoperative outcomes for pediatric patients with perforated appendicitis. Medicine. 2017;96:e8849.
11. van Rossem C, Schreinemacher M, van Geloven A, Bemelman W. Antibiotic duration after laparoscopic appendectomy for acute complicated appendicitis. JAMA Surg. 2016;151:323.
12. Rangel S, Anderson B, Srivastava R, et al. Intravenous versus oral antibiotics for the prevention of treatment failure in children with complicated appendicitis. Ann Surg. 2017;266:361–8.
13. Assarsson J, Körner U, Lundholm K. Evaluation of procalcitonin as a marker to predict antibiotic response in adult patients with acute appendicitis: a prospective observational study. Surg Infect. 2014;15:601–5.
14. Slieker J, Aellen S, Eggimann P, Guarnero V, Schäfer M, Demartines N. Procalcitonin-guided antibiotics after surgery for peritonitis: a randomized controlled study. Gastroenterol Res Pract. 2017;2017:1–6.
15. Park H, Kim M, Lee B. Randomized clinical trial of antibiotic therapy for uncomplicated appendicitis. Br J Surg. 2017;104:1785–179.
16. Kessler U, Mosbahi S, Walker B, Hau E, Cotton M, Peiry B, Berger S, Egger B. Conservative treatment versus surgery for uncomplicated appendicitis in children: a systematic review and meta-analysis. Arch Dis Child. 2017;102:1118–24.
17. Kim D, Nassiri N, Saltzman D, et al. Postoperative antibiotics are not associated with decreased wound complications among patients undergoing appendectomy for complicated appendicitis. Am J Surg. 2015;210:983–9.

Non-operative Management of Uncomplicated Appendicitis

Leo Andrew Benedict and Shawn D. St. Peter

Case Example

A 13-year-old boy presents with a 1 day history of abdominal pain that localized to the right lower quadrant. On physical exam he has signs and symptoms consistent with acute appendicitis. His laboratories reveal a white blood cell count of 12,000 per cubic millimeter of blood. He has an ultrasound performed which does not show any evidence of perforation, and no fecalith is visualized. The family asks whether there is an alternative to surgical appendectomy.

Introduction

Appendicitis remains the most common surgical emergency in children with a lifetime risk of 7–8% and a peak incidence in the teenage years [1]. In the United States, the standard of care for children diagnosed with acute appendicitis is to perform a laparoscopic appendectomy. Approximately 60,000 and 80,000 pediatric appendectomies are performed each year, with an average cost of approximately $9000 [2]. The morbidity rate varies from 5% to 30%, with higher rates reported in cases of perforated appendicitis [3–6], defined as either a hole in the appendix or a fecalith in the abdomen during the operation [7]. Major complications associated with an appendectomy include surgical site and organ-space surgical site infections, adhesive small bowel obstruction, hospital readmissions, and reoperation. Minor complications include superficial surgical site infections, urinary retention, and urinary tract infections. Efforts to avoid both major and minor complications associated with appendectomy include the use of antibiotics to manage children with uncomplicated appendicitis. There has been growing evidence regarding the use of

L. A. Benedict · S. D. St. Peter (✉)
Children's Mercy Hospital, Kansas City, MO, USA
e-mail: sspeter@cmh.edu

© Springer Nature Switzerland AG 2019
C. J. Hunter (ed.), *Controversies in Pediatric Appendicitis*,
https://doi.org/10.1007/978-3-030-15006-8_7

non-operative management (NOM) for both adults and children with uncomplicated appendicitis. In this chapter, we will review the current evidence for NOM in children.

Discussion

Managing children diagnosed with uncomplicated appendicitis without an appendectomy is a treatment option that has gained significant traction in the past few years among both providers and patient families. Despite the relatively low-risk implications of performing an appendectomy, it requires general anesthesia and is an abdominal operation with inherent risks. Complications related to surgery or anesthesia occur in more than 10% of children within 30 days of appendectomy [8]. Even with current imaging methods, 6.3% of children in Canada and 4.3% in the United States undergoing appendectomy are subsequently found to have a normal appendix [9].

Several adult trials demonstrate the benefit of using NOM for non-perforated appendicitis [10–16]. These trials show the early success rate of NOM to be approximately 90%. However, this falls to approximately 70% at 1 year, with the risk thereafter unknown [17]. These studies demonstrate similar rates of perforation and fewer complications when compared to patients undergoing an appendectomy. Furthermore, patients undergoing NOM exhibit improved pain control, shorter sick leave, but increased recurrence rates when compared to initial appendectomy [17, 18]. A recent systematic review and meta-analysis found a longer hospitalization stay with antibiotic treatment but also found an incidental malignancy rate of 0.6% [17]. While this is a lower concern in children, it still exists as we have documented an unsuspected carcinoid in 0.2% of appendectomy specimens in children [19]. The adult literature has identified several predictors for failure of NOM. These include the presence of an appendicolith, a phlegmon or abscess on imaging, an elevated white blood cell (WBC) count >18,000 or CRP >4 mg/dl, and abdominal pain for more than 48 hours [10–16]. Adult patients wishing to undergo NOM for acute appendicitis with any of these predictors should be counseled on the increased failure rate.

In children with appendicitis, the literature is a little less mature for NOM (Table 7.1) [20–29]. A pilot randomized trial performed in Sweden included 26 operative patients and 24 non-operative patients and showed a success rate of 92% at discharge and 62% at 1 year [27]. Furthermore, at 1 year follow-up, there was no increased risk of complications and similar costs among children managed nonoperatively. A second trial published from Japan was a patient choice trial from 2007 to 2013 in which 78 patients chose NOM and 86 patients elected to undergo surgery [28]. With a median follow-up of 4.3 years, the success rate for NOM was 99% at discharge and 71% at median follow-up. However, 29% of patients electing for NOM had a recurrence at 1 year. There was no difference in the operative time or rates of postoperative complications between the two groups. In a feasibility study, 24 patients between the ages of 5 and 18 years old with less than 48 hours of symptoms were enrolled and compared to 50 controls [23]. At an average follow-up of 14 months, 3 of the 24 patients failed on NOM, and 2 of 21 patients returned with

Table 7.1 Existing literature for non-operative management of acute uncomplicated appendicitis in children

Study	Year of publication	Study design	Children enrolled in non-operative management
Minneci et al.	2016	Prospective parent preference-based trial	30
Hartwich et al.	2016	Prospective parent preference-based feasibility trial	24
Tanaka et al.	2015	Non-randomized retrospective cohort	78
Steiner et al.	2015	Non-randomized prospective cohort	45
Svensson et al.	2015	Pilot randomized control trial	24
Gorter et al.	2015	Non-randomized prospective cohort	25
Koike et al.	2014	Retrospective cohort	130
Armstrong et al.	2014	Non-randomized retrospective cohort	12
Abes et al.	2007	Retrospective cohort	16
Kaneko et al.	2004	Prospective cohort	22

recurrent appendicitis at 43 and 52 days, respectively. Furthermore, two patients elected to undergo an interval appendectomy despite the absence of symptoms. The appendectomy-free rate at 1 year was 71% with no patient developing perforation or other complications. The hospital costs from this study decreased from $4130 to $2771 [23].

Finally, a prospective single-institution patient choice trial was performed in the United States that enrolled 102 children who met specific clinical inclusion criteria [26, 30]. These criteria were 7–18 years of age, less than 48 hours of abdominal pain, WBC less than 18,000 cells per microliter, and US or computed tomography (CT) scan identifying an appendix less than 1.2 cm in diameter without an appendicolith, abscess, or phlegmon. If a patient decides to undergo surgery, they receive an urgent laparoscopic appendectomy. Patients who chose non-operative management were hospitalized for at least 24 hours to receive intravenous antibiotics. They were given a diet after 12 hours; if at 24 hours they had no clinical improvement, they underwent laparoscopic appendectomy. Of the 102 enrolled patients, 65 elected for surgery, and 37 elected for NOM with antibiotics alone. The success rate for NOM was 93% at hospital discharge, 90% at 30-day follow-up, and 76% at 1 year [30]. In analyzing quality-of-life scores at 30 days, patients treated with NOM reported higher scores and fewer disability days. Furthermore, the authors demonstrated lower overall costs, no treatment-related complications, or rates of complicated appendicitis at 1 year for patients electing for NOM. The patient preference design has been expanded through the Midwest Pediatric Surgery Consortium to enroll 1000 patients in a funded trial.

Based on the previously described studies [27, 30], there is currently an international, multicenter, randomized trial to evaluate NOM for children with acute appendicitis (Fig. 7.1). This ongoing trial across 12 children's hospital in the United States, Canada, and Europe will be the largest randomized study to evaluate antibiotic treatment of acute appendicitis in children. In this trial, the inclusion criteria are age 5–16 years old, clinical and/or radiological diagnosis (US and/or CT scan) of

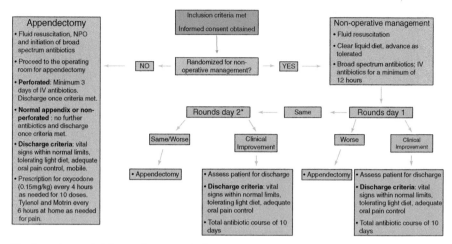

Fig. 7.1 Clinical flowchart for the current international, multicenter, randomized trial to evaluate the non-operative management for children with acute appendicitis

acute non-perforated appendicitis, and written informed parental consent. Exclusion criteria include presentation with an appendiceal mass or phlegmon (on physical examination and/or imaging), suspicion of perforated appendicitis, NOM (two or more doses of IV antibiotics) initiated at an outside institution, previous episode of appendicitis treated non-operatively, positive pregnancy test, diagnosis of cystic fibrosis, and current treatment for malignancy.

The ability to establish risk factors for failure of NOM remains essential for appropriate patient selection. Published reports in the literature suggest that an appendicolith is an adverse indicator for successful NOM [31, 32]. A prospective study evaluating the utility of NOM in children with acute appendicitis identified 47% (9/19) of patients with an appendicolith failing NOM compared to 24% (14/59) of patients without an appendicolith ($p = 0.05$) [28]. Furthermore, a small prospective, nonrandomized trial in children aged 7–17 years old was terminated early because 60% (3/5) of patients with an appendicolith failed NOM at a median follow-up of 5 months [32]. These findings indicate that parents or caregivers considering NOM for their child with an appendicolith should be educated on the reported failure rates. The available data does suggest that antibiotics alone for children found with an appendicolith on imaging may not be effective for treating acute appendicitis.

Misconceptions from both parents and caregivers that a delay in performing an appendectomy leads to a greater likelihood of developing perforated appendicitis have challenged the framework for NOM [33]. However, it has been shown that delaying appendectomy doesn't increase the risk of complications [34]. Furthermore, the increased public awareness of NOM for children with acute appendicitis is slowly improving, and we expect this treatment modality to gain significant traction as more studies show its benefit.

A second challenge for NOM in children with acute appendicitis relates to parents and caregivers developing a clear understanding of the disease process in order to make an informed management decision. A published feasibility study which included 100 participants highlighted the knowledge gap regarding the perception of appendicitis. Caregivers and patients greater than 15 years of age were questioned before and after an education session about their understanding of appendicitis. Eighty-two percent of participants thought it was likely or very likely that the appendix would rupture if the operation was delayed. In addition, the participants also acknowledged that a rupture of the appendix would lead to severe complications and even death. This study highlights the importance of patient and caregiver education which will improve the capacity to make decisions on alternative treatments for acute appendicitis [33].

The major limitation of the data on NOM is the inadequate long-term follow-up for children, making it difficult to fully assess the failure rate. Furthermore, many of the studies evaluating NOM for children with acute appendicitis have a variable duration of antibiotic therapy and length of hospital stay. To counteract these limitations, future cohort studies and prospective clinical trials need to establish core parameters during the study period so that clinical outcomes can be universally measured for comparison.

Conclusion

Based on the current body of literature utilizing the non-operative approach for children with acute uncomplicated appendicitis, the use of antibiotics is a reasonable treatment alternative to surgery in well-selected patients. Parents and caregivers should be educated on the potential benefits and risks for this approach. In addition, providers should be fully aware of the risk factors that increase the failure rate for NOM.

Clinical Pearls

- NOM of uncomplicated appendicitis appears to be a reasonable alternative to surgery in select patients.
- The presence of a fecalith or elevated laboratories is associated with a lower likelihood of successful NOM.
- Caregiver and patient family education regarding the pathophysiology of appendicitis are crucial prior to recommending NOM.

References

1. Rentea RM, St Peter SD. Pediatric appendicitis. Surg Clin North Am. 2017;97(1):93–112.
2. MacFie J, O'Boyle C, Mitchell CJ, Buckley PM, Johnstone D, Sudworth P. Gut origin of sepsis: a prospective study investigating associations between bacterial translocation, gastric microflora, and septic morbidity. Gut. 1999;45(2):223–8.

3. Ikeda H, Ishimaru Y, Takayasu H, Okamura K, Kisaki Y, Fujino J. Laparoscopic versus open appendectomy in children with uncomplicated and complicated appendicitis. J Pediatr Surg. 2004;39(11):1680–5.
4. Malagon AM, Arteaga-Gonzalez I, Rodriguez-Ballester L. Outcomes after laparoscopic treatment of complicated versus uncomplicated acute appendicitis: a prospective, comparative trial. J Laparoendosc Adv Surg Tech A. 2009;19(6):721–5.
5. Cash CL, Frazee RC, Smith RW, Davis ML, Hendricks JC, Childs EW, et al. Outpatient laparoscopic appendectomy for acute appendicitis. Am Surg. 2012;78(2):213–5.
6. Tiwari MM, Reynoso JF, Tsang AW, Oleynikov D. Comparison of outcomes of laparoscopic and open appendectomy in management of uncomplicated and complicated appendicitis. Ann Surg. 2011;254(6):927–32.
7. St Peter SD, Sharp SW, Holcomb GW 3rd, Ostlie DJ. An evidence-based definition for perforated appendicitis derived from a prospective randomized trial. J Pediatr Surg. 2008;43(12):2242–5.
8. Tiboni S, Bhangu A, Hall NJ. Paediatric surgery trainees research N, the National Surgical Research C. Outcome of appendicectomy in children performed in paediatric surgery units compared with general surgery units. Br J Surg. 2014;101(6):707–14.
9. Cheong LH, Emil S. Outcomes of pediatric appendicitis: an international comparison of the United States and Canada. JAMA Surg. 2014;149(1):50–5.
10. Di Saverio S, Sibilio A, Giorgini E, Biscardi A, Villani S, Coccolini F, et al. The NOTA Study (Non Operative Treatment for Acute Appendicitis): prospective study on the efficacy and safety of antibiotics (amoxicillin and clavulanic acid) for treating patients with right lower quadrant abdominal pain and long-term follow-up of conservatively treated suspected appendicitis. Ann Surg. 2014;260(1):109–17.
11. Hansson J, Korner U, Khorram-Manesh A, Solberg A, Lundholm K. Randomized clinical trial of antibiotic therapy versus appendicectomy as primary treatment of acute appendicitis in unselected patients. Br J Surg. 2009;96(5):473–81.
12. Shindoh J, Niwa H, Kawai K, Ohata K, Ishihara Y, Takabayashi N, et al. Predictive factors for negative outcomes in initial non-operative management of suspected appendicitis. J Gastrointest Surg. 2010;14(2):309–14.
13. Styrud J, Eriksson S, Nilsson I, Ahlberg G, Haapaniemi S, Neovius G, et al. Appendectomy versus antibiotic treatment in acute appendicitis. A prospective multicenter randomized controlled trial. World J Surg. 2006;30(6):1033–7.
14. Hansson J, Korner U, Ludwigs K, Johnsson E, Jonsson C, Lundholm K. Antibiotics as first-line therapy for acute appendicitis: evidence for a change in clinical practice. World J Surg. 2012;36(9):2028–36.
15. Salminen P, Paajanen H, Rautio T, Nordstrom P, Aarnio M, Rantanen T, et al. Antibiotic therapy vs appendectomy for treatment of uncomplicated acute appendicitis: the APPAC randomized clinical trial. JAMA. 2015;313(23):2340–8.
16. Vons C, Barry C, Maitre S, Pautrat K, Leconte M, Costaglioli B, et al. Amoxicillin plus clavulanic acid versus appendicectomy for treatment of acute uncomplicated appendicitis: an open-label, non-inferiority, randomised controlled trial. Lancet. 2011;377(9777):1573–9.
17. Findlay JM, Kafsi JE, Hammer C, Gilmour J, Gillies RS, Maynard ND. Nonoperative management of appendicitis in adults: a systematic review and meta-analysis of randomized controlled trials. J Am Coll Surg. 2016;223(6):814–24 e2.
18. Mason RJ, Moazzez A, Sohn H, Katkhouda N. Meta-analysis of randomized trials comparing antibiotic therapy with appendectomy for acute uncomplicated (no abscess or phlegmon) appendicitis. Surg Infect. 2012;13(2):74–84.
19. Alemayehu H, Snyder CL, St Peter SD, Ostlie DJ. Incidence and outcomes of unexpected pathology findings after appendectomy. J Pediatr Surg. 2014;49(9):1390–3.
20. Abes M, Petik B, Kazil S. Nonoperative treatment of acute appendicitis in children. J Pediatr Surg. 2007;42(8):1439–42.
21. Armstrong J, Merritt N, Jones S, Scott L, Butter A. Non-operative management of early, acute appendicitis in children: is it safe and effective? J Pediatr Surg. 2014;49(5):782–5.

22. Gorter RR, van der Lee JH, Cense HA, Kneepkens CM, Wijnen MH, In 't Hof KH, et al. Initial antibiotic treatment for acute simple appendicitis in children is safe: short-term results from a multicenter, prospective cohort study. Surgery. 2015;157(5):916–23.
23. Hartwich J, Luks FI, Watson-Smith D, Kurkchubasche AG, Muratore CS, Wills HE, et al. Nonoperative treatment of acute appendicitis in children: a feasibility study. J Pediatr Surg. 2016;51(1):111–6.
24. Kaneko K, Tsuda M. Ultrasound-based decision making in the treatment of acute appendicitis in children. J Pediatr Surg. 2004;39(9):1316–20.
25. Koike Y, Uchida K, Matsushita K, Otake K, Nakazawa M, Inoue M, et al. Intraluminal appendiceal fluid is a predictive factor for recurrent appendicitis after initial successful non-operative management of uncomplicated appendicitis in pediatric patients. J Pediatr Surg. 2014;49(7):1116–21.
26. Minneci PC, Mahida JB, Lodwick DL, Sulkowski JP, Nacion KM, Cooper JN, et al. Effectiveness of patient choice in nonoperative vs surgical management of pediatric uncomplicated acute appendicitis. JAMA Surg. 2016;151(5):408–15.
27. Svensson JF, Patkova B, Almstrom M, Naji H, Hall NJ, Eaton S, et al. Nonoperative treatment with antibiotics versus surgery for acute nonperforated appendicitis in children: a pilot randomized controlled trial. Ann Surg. 2015;261(1):67–71.
28. Tanaka Y, Uchida H, Kawashima H, Fujiogi M, Takazawa S, Deie K, et al. Long-term outcomes of operative versus nonoperative treatment for uncomplicated appendicitis. J Pediatr Surg. 2015;50(11):1893–7.
29. Steiner Z, Buklan G, Stackievicz R, Gutermacher M, Erez I. A role for conservative antibiotic treatment in early appendicitis in children. J Pediatr Surg. 2015;50(9):1566–8.
30. Minneci PC, Sulkowski JP, Nacion KM, Mahida JB, Cooper JN, Moss RL, et al. Feasibility of a nonoperative management strategy for uncomplicated acute appendicitis in children. J Am Coll Surg. 2014;219(2):272–9.
31. Aprahamian CJ, Barnhart DC, Bledsoe SE, Vaid Y, Harmon CM. Failure in the nonoperative management of pediatric ruptured appendicitis: predictors and consequences. J Pediatr Surg. 2007;42(6):934–8; discussion 8.
32. Mahida JB, Lodwick DL, Nacion KM, Sulkowski JP, Leonhart KL, Cooper JN, et al. High failure rate of nonoperative management of acute appendicitis with an appendicolith in children. J Pediatr Surg. 2016;51(6):908–11.
33. Chau DB, Ciullo SS, Watson-Smith D, Chun TH, Kurkchubasche AG, Luks FI. Patient-centered outcomes research in appendicitis in children: bridging the knowledge gap. J Pediatr Surg. 2016;51(1):117–21.
34. Boomer LA, Cooper JN, Anandalwar S, Fallon SC, Ostlie D, Leys CM, et al. Delaying appendectomy does not lead to higher rates of surgical site infections: a multi-institutional analysis of children with appendicitis. Ann Surg. 2016;264(1):164–8.

Non-operative Management of Complicated Appendicitis

Emily D. Dubina and Steven L. Lee

Case Example

A 10-year-old girl presents to the emergency department with her parents complaining of 5 days of right lower quadrant abdominal pain. She has been intermittently febrile at home to 38.5 °C and she has a leukocytosis of 16.1×10^9/L. On examination, she is noted to have a palpable mass in the right lower quadrant, which is confirmed on ultrasound to be a 3×3 cm abscess, likely due to perforated appendicitis. She is admitted, placed on intravenous antibiotics until resolution of her fevers and improvement of her abdominal pain and leukocytosis. She is then discharged home on oral antibiotics once tolerating a diet. She is scheduled to return to clinic for evaluation for interval appendectomy.

Introduction

Acute appendicitis has a spectrum of presentations, from simple inflammation of the appendix to perforation with gross fecal contamination. Complicated appendicitis itself includes a wide spectrum, from gangrenous to perforated, with the possibility of the development of an associated phlegmon or abscess or with diffuse peritonitis. The incidence of perforated appendicitis in the pediatric population is approximately 30% [1]; this number has even been estimated as high as 38.7% in other studies, with the finding that up to 65.8% of pediatric patients under age 4 years will present with perforation [2]. Once perforated, the course of care is complicated by a longer length of stay, longer duration of antibiotics, and greater

E. D. Dubina
Department of Surgery, Harbor-UCLA Medical Center, Torrance, CA, USA

S. L. Lee (✉)
Division of Pediatric Surgery, Mattel Children's Hospital at the University of California, Los Angeles Medical Center, Westwood, CA, USA

© Springer Nature Switzerland AG 2019
C. J. Hunter (ed.), *Controversies in Pediatric Appendicitis*,
https://doi.org/10.1007/978-3-030-15006-8_8

financial expense as compared to non-complicated acute appendicitis [2]. In addition to the variable course of complicated appendicitis, there is significant provider variability in the management of this disease process. Multiple studies have described the benefits of early appendectomy, even in the setting of complicated appendicitis [3–13]. However, non-operative therapy can also be effective in the management of complicated appendicitis and in certain circumstances should be the preferred approach. In this chapter, we will explore the non-operative management of complicated pediatric appendicitis and provide treatment recommendations for practice.

The Role for Non-operative Management

The optimal treatment of complicated appendicitis (gangrenous or perforated plus or minus an associated phlegmon or abscess) remains controversial. A 1981 study by Jordan et al. of 45 patients presenting with an abdominal or pelvic mass with appendicitis demonstrated a 33.7% complication rate in the 90.5% of patients who underwent appendectomy within 24 hours of admission (primarily wound infections) [3]. Despite this, multiple studies are in support of early appendectomy, even in patients presenting with complicated appendicitis who are at higher risk of complications. Blakely et al., in a 2011 study of 131 patients with perforated appendicitis without mass or abscess, randomized patients to early appendectomy (within 24 hours of admission) versus initial non-operative management with interval appendectomy (within 6–8 weeks); they found adverse events in 30% of early appendectomy patients as compared to 55% of interval appendectomy patients, as well as a reduced time away from normal activities for early appendectomy patients in addition to a 34% failure rate for patients randomized to the interval appendectomy group due to failure to improve or recurrent symptoms of acute appendicitis [5]. In light of these findings, they suggested that early appendectomy was better than non-operative management with interval appendectomy [5]. The results of this single randomized trial have dominated the recommendations of multiple meta-analysis studies and led to the recommendation of early appendectomy for complicated appendicitis [9, 10]. Retrospective reviews have also found that early appendectomy is associated with decreased length of stay, morbidity, and overall complications [4, 7, 8, 12, 13], as well as lower hospital costs and healthcare utilization as compared to non-operative management with interval appendectomy [6, 11].

Despite the findings of these studies, there has also been ample evidence to support a trial of non-operative management for complicated appendicitis in certain patients. As early as 1980, Janik et al. described an ultraconservative approach to non-operative management of late-presenting complicated appendicitis in which 37 children were observed in the hospital without antibiotic management until they had improvement in symptoms; 81% of the children demonstrated clinical improvement in 5–22 days, and only 19% required abscess drainage within 2–10 days of presentation, with only 1 child presenting with recurrent symptoms [14]. They concluded that non-operative management without antibiotics is safe with close observation and that interval appendectomy can be performed up to 20 weeks after symptom resolution [14]. In 1981, Powers et al. described non-operative or conservative management of perforated appendicitis with interval appendectomy 4–6 weeks later if there was good clinical response and described good safety with this approach; however, they cautioned that if there was no clinical improvement on antibiotics within 12–24 hours, then appendectomy was indicated at that time [15]. Skoubo-Kristensen and Hvid, in 1982, described a series of 193 adult and pediatric patients with an appendiceal mass or abscess treated over a period of 10 years with non-operative management; they found an 88% success rate with non-operative management, with a 7.1% recurrence rate over a 3-month period [16]. They felt that patients presenting with appendicitis with an appendiceal mass were successful in most patients, with low complication rates for interval appendectomy [16]. In 1987, Bagi and Dueholm described using non-operative management with intravenous antibiotics and percutaneous drainage if there was a verified abscess which could be safely drained for patients presenting with appendicitis with an appendiceal mass [17]. They found that non-operative management was safe, with relatively few complications or late sequelae; patients do, however, require close monitoring upon discharge [17].

These early studies laid the groundwork for future work describing successful non-operative management of complicated appendicitis. One aspect to consider is whether the patient is presenting simply with a perforated appendicitis or whether they are presenting with a perforated appendicitis with a well-formed appendiceal mass or abscess. A number of studies have examined the success of conservative management with initial intravenous antibiotics with the addition of percutaneous drainage if possible in the treatment of perforated appendicitis with a well-defined abscess or mass [18–29]. In a large study of 427 children presenting with abdominal mass with appendicitis at three children's hospitals, 16 underwent immediate appendectomy and 411 were treated conservatively; the authors described an 84.2% success rate of initial non-operative management, with a median length of stay of 6 days. The complication rate following interval appendectomy 4–6 weeks later was only 2.3% [19]. Roach et al., in a study of 92 pediatric patients with complicated appendicitis and an intra-abdominal abscess or phlegmon, where 60 were taken immediately to the operating room and 32 were treated with intravenous antibiotics and abscess drainage followed by interval appendectomy around 6 weeks later, found that the conservative management group demonstrated no difference in length of stay and no readmissions, while there were 6 readmissions in the immediate operation group; they concluded that patients presenting with more than 5 days of symptoms with a well-defined mass or abscess could be successfully treated with antibiotics and drainage when possible [22]. These and other similar studies support the use of non-operative management for pediatric patients presenting with appendicitis with an associated appendiceal mass or abscess, with good success rates and minimal complications as compared to those patients undergoing immediate or early appendectomy.

The success of non-operative management extends beyond the treatment of patients presenting with appendiceal mass or abscess, however. Successful non-operative management has also been described in groups of patients presenting with complicated appendicitis with no distinction based on the presence or absence of appendiceal mass or abscess [30–36], as well as in mixed populations of patients presenting with and without abscess or mass [37–40]. A 2003 study of 96 children being treated for perforated appendicitis, where 71 underwent immediate appendectomy and 25 were treated initially non-operatively with antibiotics and percutaneous drainage if necessary, demonstrated a success rate of 64%; however, in the 9 children who required earlier appendectomy (after 3–12 days), those patients had fewer wound complications and abscesses postoperatively compared to those patients undergoing immediate appendectomy, therefore favoring initial delayed or non-operative management [37]. Vane and Fernandez compared 86 children presenting with complicated appendicitis based on those undergoing immediate appendectomy within 72 hours (59 children) and those undergoing initial non-operative management with interval appendectomy (27 children); they found that the length of stay was 4.9 days for the immediate group and 4.1 days for the interval group plus an additional 0.9 days for the interval appendectomy and that all of the complications occurred in the immediate appendectomy group, further supporting the use of non-operative management in complicated appendicitis [31]. In a 2013 study of children presenting with complicated appendicitis being treated non-operatively, the authors expanded the criteria for non-operative management to include almost anyone beyond those presenting with simple appendicitis; they found the average length of stay to be 5.6 days, and only 4.9% required appendectomy prior to discharge for failure to improve [40]. In a meta-analysis comparing conservative treatment of complicated appendicitis versus immediate appendectomy, Simillis et al. looked specifically at studies pertaining to the pediatric population and demonstrated that as compared to conservative management, pediatric patients undergoing immediate appendectomy had more complications, including wound infections and intra-abdominal abscesses, with no difference in the initial length of stay, the rate of ileus or small bowel obstruction, or the need for reoperations; this large meta-analysis further supports the use of non-operative management in pediatric patients presenting with complicated appendicitis [41]. All of these studies taken together support a careful use of a trial of initial non-operative management, including intravenous fluid resuscitation, intravenous antibiotics, and percutaneous drainage if possible for complicated appendicitis, regardless of whether or not there is a well-formed abscess or mass at the time of presentation.

The Cost of Non-operative Management

When comparing initial non-operative management to early appendectomy, the hospital-related costs must also be taken into account. The majority of studies report that early appendectomy is associated with decreased costs as compared to interval appendectomy following non-operative management [6, 8, 11, 24, 42]. A study by Darwazeh et al. in 2016 found that interval appendectomy prevents a recurrence in only one of eight patients (pediatric and adult); therefore significant additional operative costs are being used for a diminishing return [42]. Dennett found that while the total hospital costs were greater for the non-operative management group, the indirect costs to patients and their families were not significantly greater [8]. While Keckler et al. support a trial of non-operative management with antibiotics and possible percutaneous drainage, they did advise that this treatment methodology can be related to an increased number of visits, and increased CT scans, leading to overall increased costs [24].

One author encouraged continued non-operative management instead of interval appendectomy if the non-operative success rate is estimated to be 60% or greater, as the potential costs of repeat admissions and procedures did not outweigh the cost associated with routine interval appendectomies [43]. Similarly, a 2014 study questioned the usefulness of routine interval appendectomy, as only 12% of patients in the study developed recurrent appendicitis, and this could lead to significant potential cost savings [26].

The Role for Patient Selection in Non-operative Management

Proper patient selection for non-operative management is key to its success. Patients presenting with diffuse peritonitis or a short duration of symptoms are typically better served by early operative management [4, 23, 38, 44]. However, those patients presenting with a longer duration of symptoms (typically greater than 5 days) and no diffuse peritonitis may be candidates for non-operative management [22, 23]. Additionally, those patients presenting with a palpable mass or visualized abscess on imaging are typically better candidates for non-operative management [45].

The key to successful non-operative management is to attempt to identify those patients who will likely fail non-operative management early in the course of their treatment. Multiple studies have been done to attempt to identify risk factors which may contribute to the failure of non-operative management [34, 35, 38, 39, 45–48]. In a 2001 study, Kogut et al. found that 22% of children being treated non-operatively for perforated appendicitis failed to improve on antibiotics and went on to appendectomy; they found that the white count differential, and in particular bandemia >15%, was correlated with treatment failure and future complications [47]. Talishinskiy et al. similarly found that bandemia >15% was associated with non-operative treatment failure [35], and Whyte et al. demonstrated that a higher percentage of bands on admission white count differential was predictive of failure [48]. The presence of an appendicolith on initial imaging is also predictive of treatment failure, as described in multiple studies [25, 34, 44, 46]. In a 2005 study, Ein et al. described a recurrence rate of 72% for patients with an appendicolith, as compared to 26% with no appendicolith [44]. Nazarey et al. described the presence of an appendicolith along with a leukocytosis >15, or patients presenting with more than 2 days of symptoms, was associated with treatment failure [34]. Zhang et al., interestingly, found that not all patients with an appendicolith on initial imaging failed non-operative therapy, as most appendicoliths which are present on the admission imaging will resolve; however, if the appendicolith persists on subsequent imaging, this is a risk factor for non-operative treatment failure [25]. Other predictors of non-operative treatment failure include lack of an abscess on admission imaging [46], evidence of disease extension beyond the right lower quadrant on admission imaging [39], requiring percutaneous drainage of an intra-abdominal abscess [38], and lack of fever response within 24 hours of initiation of treatment [48]. If these risk factors are not present, it is possible that patients will have greater success with non-operative management. It is important to make the decision early in the patient's presentation as to whether or not they will be a good candidate for non-operative management, as failure of non-operative management can lead to significant complications.

The Role for Antibiotic Selection in Non-operative Management

While individual hospitals or providers may have their own protocols for the non-operative management of complicated appendicitis, management typically is begun with fluid resuscitation, as well as initiation of broad-spectrum antibiotics.

Multiple antibiotic regimens have been described [4, 5, 11, 12, 30, 40, 49]. The classic starting regimen of intravenous antibiotics for perforated appendicitis includes the triple therapy of ampicillin, gentamicin, and clindamycin or metronidazole [4, 31]. Studies have since demonstrated efficacy with other antibiotic combinations such as ceftriaxone and metronidazole, which is felt to be less costly with no difference in length of stay or the rate of postoperative complications [4, 50, 51], or ticarcillin/clavulanate plus gentamicin, which was found to be clinically more effective than the traditional triple therapy [4, 52]. The use of piperacillin-tazobactam plus or minus metronidazole has also been described [40, 49]. Bufo et al. in 1998 described treatment with ceftazidime and clindamycin, with a non-operative failure rate of 17% [30].

The ideal antibiotic for discharge home has also been explored. Interestingly, higher numbers of treatment failures have been identified in patients remaining on intravenous antibiotics via a peripherally inserted central catheter (PICC) line upon discharge home. The treatment failures and revisits are thought to be due in part to complications arising from the PICC line [53]. Oral antibiotics which have been used with successful discharge include amoxicillin/clavulanate with metronidazole [40] and trimethoprim-sulfamethoxazole with metronidazole [23, 31].

The Role for Percutaneous Drainage in Non-operative Management

If an abscess is identified on admission imaging or the patient has a palpable mass on physical examination, percutaneous drainage can be a valuable addition to the success of non-operative management. Even starting as early as 1987, practitioners were abdicating for non-operative management in complicated appendicitis with abscess, including percutaneous drainage of the abscess if possible [17]. A 2016 study by Luo et al. included 1225 pediatric patients with appendiceal abscess undergoing non-operative management; 150 underwent percutaneous drainage (2.2%), whereas 1075 (97.8%) were treated with antibiotics alone and no percutaneous drainage. The patients who underwent percutaneous drainage had a longer length of stay, but less recurrences and fewer complications following interval appendectomy if it was performed; the authors concluded that antibiotics plus percutaneous drainage was more effective treatment for appendiceal abscess than antibiotics alone [29]. McNeeley et al. similarly described significant symptom improvement with percutaneous drainage; however, they did find that more complicated abscesses had a higher rate of technical failure or possible subsequent recurrence or complications [54]. Roach et al., in a study of 92 pediatric patients with complicated appendicitis with intra-abdominal abscess in which 32 patients had percutaneous drainage and treatment with intravenous followed by oral antibiotics and 60 patients were taken immediately to the operating room, found that those patients undergoing non-operative management with interval appendectomy at a later date had no difference in length of stay and an improved readmission profile as compared to the immediate appendectomy group; they therefore support percutaneous drainage and interval appendectomy in patients who present with prolonged symptoms and a discrete abscess or phlegmon [22]. In a 2010 study, St. Peter et al. randomized children presenting with appendiceal abscess to early appendectomy or percutaneous drainage with antibiotics and an interval appendectomy; they found that 11 of 20 patients had successful placement of percutaneous drain, and three patients had aspiration of the abscess with no drain left (six patients had an abscess not amenable to drainage). The patients who were successfully drained had a quick return to regular diet as well as a shorter operation as compared to the early appendectomy group [55].

Depending on the size of the abscess, it is possible that no percutaneous drainage is necessary and that intravenous antibiotics alone are sufficient for treatment. In a 2013 study, Gasior et al. performed a retrospective review of 217 children presenting with appendiceal abscess with perforated appendicitis. They found that abscess less than 20 cm^2 may be successfully treated with antibiotics alone and no percutaneous drainage [56]. In a 1991 study, Hoffmann et al. described a series of 28 patients in which abscess drainage was avoided and the patients were treated with intravenous antibiotics and observation alone; there were no in-hospital complications, with a median stay of 10 days and only one patient presenting with recurrent appendicitis and one with recurrent abscess [18]. This suggests that it may be possible to treat complicated appendicitis with abscess with intravenous antibiotics alone.

The Role for Performance of Interval Appendectomy in Non-operative Management

Early supporters of non-operative management for complicated appendicitis included the recommendation for interval appendectomy anywhere from 4 to 20 weeks following resolution of acute appendicitis [14, 15]. Recent practice guidelines for perforated appendicitis found that the risk of recurrence is approximately 8–15% (or 1–3% per year) and therefore made an argument for interval appendectomy [57]. Multiple other studies have supported interval appendectomy after successful non-operative management to prevent recurrence (especially in patients with appendicolith, the presence of which significantly increases the risk of recurrent appendicitis) and to rule out other pathologies such as carcinoid tumor [19–22, 31, 33, 37, 44, 58, 59]. A handful of studies have examined the histopathology of interval appendectomy specimens and have found that the rate of an obliterated appendiceal lumen is relatively low, which leaves the patient at increased risk of recurrent appendicitis since we are unable to determine whether or not the appendix lumen is obliterated without removing the specimen surgically [20, 33, 58].

Conversely, there have been multiple studies in recent years arguing against the routine performance of interval appendectomy following successful non-operative management of complicated appendicitis for all patients. Significant findings in these studies include a low risk of recurrence [42, 60–62], the associated costs with routine interval appendectomy [6, 26, 42, 43], and a lack of superiority evidence for interval appendectomy [63], in addition to the psychosocial impact on the patient and their family [64].

Conclusions

The optimal treatment of complicated appendicitis remains controversial. Whereas clinical practice guidelines have been developed for the operative management of perforated appendicitis with the ability to decrease resource utilization and improve patient outcomes [65, 66], the same has not yet been done for the non-operative management of perforated appendicitis. See Fig. 8.1 for a recommended treatment algorithm. Patients presenting initially with a short duration of symptoms (<5 days) or diffuse peritonitis should proceed to the operating room for early appendectomy following initiation of fluid resuscitation and broad-spectrum antibiotics. If, however, there is no diffuse peritonitis on exam and symptoms have been present for >5 days, the patient is potentially a candidate for non-operative management.

Patients should be adequately resuscitated with intravenous fluids and started on broad-spectrum intravenous antibiotics (preferably ceftriaxone/flagyl) while kept initially NPO. If there is an abscess present on imaging which is >20 cm^2 and amenable to percutaneous drainage, this should be performed by interventional radiology. If there is no abscess and only phlegmon, or the abscess is <20 cm^2, treatment should continue with intravenous antibiotics alone. Close clinical monitoring is necessary at the outset of non-operative treatment to identify those patients who are failing non-operative therapy. If there is no clinical improvement (decreased abdominal pain, improving leukocytosis, reduced fevers) within the first 24–48 hours, non-operative management should be abandoned, and the patient should be taken to the operating room for appendectomy.

The duration of intravenous antibiotic therapy is based on clinical parameters. Once a patient is afebrile for at least 24 hours, his or her pain is adequately

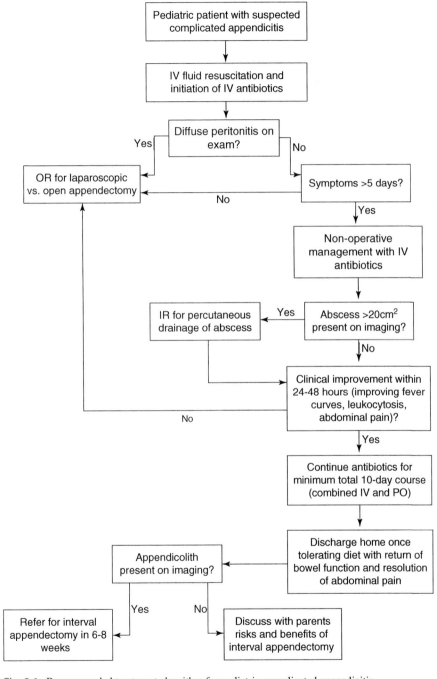

Fig. 8.1 Recommended treatment algorithm for pediatric complicated appendicitis

controlled, and he or she is tolerating a diet with normal bowel function, the patient is considered ready for discharge. The use of oral antibiotic regimens remains controversial; if administered, they should be similar in action to the intravenous regimen (such as amoxicillin/clavulanate plus metronidazole or trimethoprim-sulfamethoxazole plus metronidazole), and the total course of antibiotics (intravenous plus oral) should be 10 days.

Following successful non-operative management, patients with appendicolith should be followed up in clinic to arrange for interval appendectomy approximately 6–8 weeks after the episode of acute appendicitis; in patients with no appendicolith, a discussion should be had with the parents to discuss the risks and benefits of interval appendectomy, and the decision should be left up to them of whether or not to proceed with interval appendectomy.

Clinical Pearls

- Patients with >5 days of symptoms but without signs of peritonitis may be considered for non-operative management.
- Close clinical monitoring is necessary to ensure that patients are improving with non-operative management.
- In cases of failure of non-operative management, an operation is necessary.
- Interval appendectomy should be considered.

References

1. Barrett ML, Hines AL, Andrews RM. Trends in rates of perforated appendix, 2001–2010: statistical brief #159. In: Healthcare cost and utilization project (HCUP) statistical briefs. Rockville: Agency for Healthcare Research and Quality (US); 2006. http://www.ncbi.nlm.nih.gov/books/NBK169006/. Accessed 8 May 2018.
2. Newman K, Ponsky T, Kittle K, et al. Appendicitis 2000: variability in practice, outcomes, and resource utilization at thirty pediatric hospitals. J Pediatr Surg. 2003;38(3):372–9; discussion 372–9. https://doi.org/10.1053/jpsu.2003.50111.
3. Jordan JS, Kovalcik PJ, Schwab CW. Appendicitis with a palpable mass. Ann Surg. 1981;193(2):227–9.
4. Morrow SE, Newman KD. Current management of appendicitis. Semin Pediatr Surg. 2007;16(1):34–40. https://doi.org/10.1053/j.sempedsurg.2006.10.005.
5. Blakely ML, Williams R, Dassinger MS, et al. Early vs interval appendectomy for children with perforated appendicitis. Arch Surg Chic Ill 1960. 2011;146(6):660–5. https://doi.org/10.1001/archsurg.2011.6.
6. Myers AL, Williams RF, Giles K, et al. Hospital cost analysis of a prospective, randomized trial of early vs interval appendectomy for perforated appendicitis in children. J Am Coll Surg. 2012;214(4):427–34; discussion 434–5. https://doi.org/10.1016/j.jamcollsurg.2011.12.026.
7. Holcomb GW, St Peter SD. Current management of complicated appendicitis in children. Eur J Pediatr Surg. 2012;22(3):207–12. https://doi.org/10.1055/s-0032-1320016.
8. Dennett KV, Tracy S, Fisher S, et al. Treatment of perforated appendicitis in children: what is the cost? J Pediatr Surg. 2012;47(6):1177–84. https://doi.org/10.1016/j.jpedsurg.2012.03.024.
9. St Peter SD, Snyder CL. Operative management of appendicitis. Semin Pediatr Surg. 2016;25(4):208–11. https://doi.org/10.1053/j.sempedsurg.2016.05.003.

10. Duggan EM, Marshall AP, Weaver KL, et al. A systematic review and individual patient data meta-analysis of published randomized clinical trials comparing early versus interval appendectomy for children with perforated appendicitis. Pediatr Surg Int. 2016;32(7):649–55. https://doi.org/10.1007/s00383-016-3897-y.
11. Church JT, Klein EJ, Carr BD, Bruch SW. Early appendectomy reduces costs in children with perforated appendicitis. J Surg Res. 2017;220:119–24. https://doi.org/10.1016/j.jss.2017.07.001.
12. Bonadio W, Rebillot K, Ukwuoma O, Saracino C, Iskhakov A. Management of pediatric perforated appendicitis: comparing outcomes using early appendectomy versus solely medical management. Pediatr Infect Dis J. 2017;36(10):937–41. https://doi.org/10.1097/INF.0000000000001025.
13. Lotti M. Second date appendectomy: operating for failure of nonoperative treatment in perforated appendicitis. Am J Emerg Med. 2017;35(6):939.e3–6. https://doi.org/10.1016/j.ajem.2016.12.072.
14. Janik JS, Ein SH, Shandling B, Simpson JS, Stephens CA. Nonsurgical management of appendiceal mass in late presenting children. J Pediatr Surg. 1980;15(4):574–6.
15. Powers RJ, Andrassy RJ, Brennan LP, Weitzman JJ. Alternate approach to the management of acute perforating appendicitis in children. Surg Gynecol Obstet. 1981;152(4):473–5.
16. Skoubo-Kristensen E, Hvid I. The appendiceal mass: results of conservative management. Ann Surg. 1982;196(5):584–7.
17. Bagi P, Dueholm S. Nonoperative management of the ultrasonically evaluated appendiceal mass. Surgery. 1987;101(5):602–5.
18. Hoffmann J, Rolff M, Lomborg V, Franzmann M. Ultraconservative management of appendiceal abscess. J R Coll Surg Edinb. 1991;36(1):18–20.
19. Gillick J, Velayudham M, Puri P. Conservative management of appendix mass in children. Br J Surg. 2001;88(11):1539–42. https://doi.org/10.1046/j.0007-1323.2001.01912.x.
20. Erdoğan D, Karaman I, Narci A, et al. Comparison of two methods for the management of appendicular mass in children. Pediatr Surg Int. 2005;21(2):81–3. https://doi.org/10.1007/s00383-004-1334-0.
21. Owen A, Moore O, Marven S, Roberts J. Interval laparoscopic appendectomy in children. J Laparoendosc Adv Surg Tech A. 2006;16(3):308–11. https://doi.org/10.1089/lap.2006.16.308.
22. Roach JP, Partrick DA, Bruny JL, Allshouse MJ, Karrer FM, Ziegler MM. Complicated appendicitis in children: a clear role for drainage and delayed appendectomy. Am J Surg. 2007;194(6):769–72; discussion 772–3. https://doi.org/10.1016/j.amjsurg.2007.08.021.
23. Emil S, Duong S. Antibiotic therapy and interval appendectomy for perforated appendicitis in children: a selective approach. Am Surg. 2007;73(9):917–22.
24. Keckler SJ, Tsao K, Sharp SW, Ostlie DJ, Holcomb GW, St Peter SD. Resource utilization and outcomes from percutaneous drainage and interval appendectomy for perforated appendicitis with abscess. J Pediatr Surg. 2008;43(6):977–80. https://doi.org/10.1016/j.jpedsurg.2008.02.019.
25. Zhang H-L, Bai Y-Z, Zhou X, Wang W-L. Nonoperative management of appendiceal phlegmon or abscess with an appendicolith in children. J Gastrointest Surg. 2013;17(4):766–70. https://doi.org/10.1007/s11605-013-2143-3.
26. Fawkner-Corbett D, Jawaid WB, McPartland J, Losty PD. Interval appendectomy in children clinical outcomes, financial costs and patient benefits. Pediatr Surg Int. 2014;30(7):743–6. https://doi.org/10.1007/s00383-014-3521-y.
27. Furuya T, Inoue M, Sugito K, et al. Effectiveness of interval appendectomy after conservative treatment of pediatric ruptured appendicitis with abscess. Indian J Surg. 2015;77(Suppl 3):1041–4. https://doi.org/10.1007/s12262-014-1121-7.
28. Guida E, Pederiva F, Grazia MD, et al. Perforated appendix with abscess: immediate or interval appendectomy? Some examples to explain our choice. Int J Surg Case Rep. 2015;12:15–8. https://doi.org/10.1016/j.ijscr.2015.05.003.
29. Luo C-C, Cheng K-F, Huang C-S, et al. Therapeutic effectiveness of percutaneous drainage and factors for performing an interval appendectomy in pediatric appendiceal abscess. BMC Surg. 2016;16(1):72. https://doi.org/10.1186/s12893-016-0188-4.

30. Bufo AJ, Shah RS, Li MH, et al. Interval appendectomy for perforated appendicitis in children. J Laparoendosc Adv Surg Tech A. 1998;8(4):209–14. https://doi.org/10.1089/lap.1998.8.209.
31. Vane DW, Fernandez N. Role of interval appendectomy in the management of complicated appendicitis in children. World J Surg. 2006;30(1):51–4. https://doi.org/10.1007/s00268-005-7946-2.
32. Henry MCW, Gollin G, Islam S, et al. Matched analysis of nonoperative management vs immediate appendectomy for perforated appendicitis. J Pediatr Surg. 2007;42(1):19–23; discussion 23–4. https://doi.org/10.1016/j.jpedsurg.2006.09.005.
33. Iqbal CW, Knott EM, Mortellaro VE, Fitzgerald KM, Sharp SW, St Peter SD. Interval appendectomy after perforated appendicitis: what are the operative risks and luminal patency rates? J Surg Res. 2012;177(1):127–30. https://doi.org/10.1016/j.jss.2012.03.009.
34. Nazarey PP, Stylianos S, Velis E, et al. Treatment of suspected acute perforated appendicitis with antibiotics and interval appendectomy. J Pediatr Surg. 2014;49(3):447–50. https://doi.org/10.1016/j.jpedsurg.2013.10.001.
35. Talishinskiy T, Limberg J, Ginsburg H, Kuenzler K, Fisher J, Tomita S. Factors associated with failure of nonoperative treatment of complicated appendicitis in children. J Pediatr Surg. 2016;51(7):1174–6. https://doi.org/10.1016/j.jpedsurg.2016.01.006.
36. López JJ, Deans KJ, Minneci PC. Nonoperative management of appendicitis in children. Curr Opin Pediatr. 2017;29(3):358–62. https://doi.org/10.1097/MOP.0000000000000487.
37. Weber TR, Keller MA, Bower RJ, Spinner G, Vierling K. Is delayed operative treatment worth the trouble with perforated appendicitis is children? Am J Surg. 2003;186(6):685–8; discussion 688–9.
38. Nadler EP, Reblock KK, Vaughan KG, Meza MP, Ford HR, Gaines BA. Predictors of outcome for children with perforated appendicitis initially treated with non-operative management. Surg Infect. 2004;5(4):349–56. https://doi.org/10.1089/sur.2004.5.349.
39. Levin T, Whyte C, Borzykowski R, Han B, Blitman N, Harris B. Nonoperative management of perforated appendicitis in children: can CT predict outcome? Pediatr Radiol. 2007;37(3):251–5. https://doi.org/10.1007/s00247-006-0384-y.
40. Fawley J, Gollin G. Expanded utilization of nonoperative management for complicated appendicitis in children. Langenbeck's Arch Surg. 2013;398(3):463–6. https://doi.org/10.1007/s00423-012-1042-5.
41. Simillis C, Symeonides P, Shorthouse AJ, Tekkis PP. A meta-analysis comparing conservative treatment versus acute appendectomy for complicated appendicitis (abscess or phlegmon). Surgery. 2010;147(6):818–29. https://doi.org/10.1016/j.surg.2009.11.013.
42. Darwazeh G, Cunningham SC, Kowdley GC. A systematic review of perforated appendicitis and Phlegmon: interval appendectomy or wait-and-see? Am Surg. 2016;82(1):11–5.
43. Raval MV, Lautz T, Reynolds M, Browne M. Dollars and sense of interval appendectomy in children: a cost analysis. J Pediatr Surg. 2010;45(9):1817–25. https://doi.org/10.1016/j.jpedsurg.2010.03.016.
44. Ein SH, Langer JC, Daneman A. Nonoperative management of pediatric ruptured appendix with inflammatory mass or abscess: presence of an appendicolith predicts recurrent appendicitis. J Pediatr Surg. 2005;40(10):1612–5. https://doi.org/10.1016/j.jpedsurg.2005.06.001.
45. Gonzalez DO, Deans KJ, Minneci PC. Role of non-operative management in pediatric appendicitis. Semin Pediatr Surg. 2016;25(4):204–7. https://doi.org/10.1053/j.sempedsurg.2016.05.002.
46. Aprahamian CJ, Barnhart DC, Bledsoe SE, Vaid Y, Harmon CM. Failure in the nonoperative management of pediatric ruptured appendicitis: predictors and consequences. J Pediatr Surg. 2007;42(6):934–8; discussion 938. https://doi.org/10.1016/j.jpedsurg.2007.01.024.
47. Kogut KA, Blakely ML, Schropp KP, et al. The association of elevated percent bands on admission with failure and complications of interval appendectomy. J Pediatr Surg. 2001;36(1):165–8.
48. Whyte C, Levin T, Harris BH. Early decisions in perforated appendicitis in children: lessons from a study of nonoperative management. J Pediatr Surg. 2008;43(8):1459–63. https://doi.org/10.1016/j.jpedsurg.2007.11.032.

49. Fishman SJ, Pelosi L, Klavon SL, O'Rourke EJ. Perforated appendicitis: prospective outcome analysis for 150 children. J Pediatr Surg. 2000;35(6):923–6. https://doi.org/10.1053/jpsu.2000.6924.
50. Hurst AL, Olson D, Somme S, et al. Once-daily ceftriaxone plus metronidazole versus ertapenem and/or cefoxitin for pediatric appendicitis. J Pediatr Infect Dis Soc. 2017;6(1):57–64. https://doi.org/10.1093/jpids/piv082.
51. St Peter SD, Little DC, Calkins CM, et al. A simple and more cost-effective antibiotic regimen for perforated appendicitis. J Pediatr Surg. 2006;41(5):1020–4. https://doi.org/10.1016/j.jpedsurg.2005.12.054.
52. Rodriguez JC, Buckner D, Schoenike S, Gomez-Marin O, Oiticica C, Thompson WR. Comparison of two antibiotic regimens in the treatment of perforated appendicitis in pediatric patients. Int J Clin Pharmacol Ther. 2000;38(10):492–9.
53. Rangel SJ, Anderson BR, Srivastava R, et al. Intravenous versus oral antibiotics for the prevention of treatment failure in children with complicated appendicitis: has the abandonment of peripherally inserted catheters been justified? Ann Surg. 2017;266(2):361–8. https://doi.org/10.1097/SLA.0000000000001923.
54. McNeeley MF, Vo NJ, Prabhu SJ, Vergnani J, Shaw DW. Percutaneous drainage of intraabdominal abscess in children with perforated appendicitis. Pediatr Radiol. 2012;42(7):805–12. https://doi.org/10.1007/s00247-011-2337-3.
55. St Peter SD, Aguayo P, Fraser JD, et al. Initial laparoscopic appendectomy versus initial nonoperative management and interval appendectomy for perforated appendicitis with abscess: a prospective, randomized trial. J Pediatr Surg. 2010;45(1):236–40. https://doi.org/10.1016/j.jpedsurg.2009.10.039.
56. Gasior AC, Marty Knott E, Ostlie DJ, St Peter SD. To drain or not to drain: an analysis of abscess drains in the treatment of appendicitis with abscess. Pediatr Surg Int. 2013;29(5):455–8. https://doi.org/10.1007/s00383-013-3262-3.
57. Rentea RM, St Peter SD. Pediatric appendicitis. Surg Clin North Am. 2017;97(1):93–112. https://doi.org/10.1016/j.suc.2016.08.009.
58. Gahukamble DB, Gahukamble LD. Surgical and pathological basis for interval appendicectomy after resolution of appendicular mass in children. J Pediatr Surg. 2000;35(3):424–7.
59. Vargas HI, Averbook A, Stamos MJ. Appendiceal mass: conservative therapy followed by interval laparoscopic appendectomy. Am Surg. 1994;60(10):753–8.
60. Puapong D, Lee SL, Haigh PI, Kaminski A, Liu I-LA, Applebaum H. Routine interval appendectomy in children is not indicated. J Pediatr Surg. 2007;42(9):1500–3. https://doi.org/10.1016/j.jpedsurg.2007.04.011.
61. Hall NJ, Jones CE, Eaton S, Stanton MP, Burge DM. Is interval appendicectomy justified after successful nonoperative treatment of an appendix mass in children? A systematic review. J Pediatr Surg. 2011;46(4):767–71. https://doi.org/10.1016/j.jpedsurg.2011.01.019.
62. Kaminski A, Liu I-LA, Applebaum H, Lee SL, Haigh PI. Routine interval appendectomy is not justified after initial nonoperative treatment of acute appendicitis. Arch Surg Chic Ill 1960. 2005;140(9):897–901.
63. Tanaka Y, Uchida H, Kawashima H, et al. More than one-third of successfully nonoperatively treated patients with complicated appendicitis experienced recurrent appendicitis: is interval appendectomy necessary? J Pediatr Surg. 2016;51(12):1957–61. https://doi.org/10.1016/j.jpedsurg.2016.09.017.
64. Schurman JV, Cushing CC, Garey CL, Laituri CA, St Peter SD. Quality of life assessment between laparoscopic appendectomy at presentation and interval appendectomy for perforated appendicitis with abscess: analysis of a prospective randomized trial. J Pediatr Surg. 2011;46(6):1121–5. https://doi.org/10.1016/j.jpedsurg.2011.03.038.
65. Willis ZI, Duggan EM, Bucher BT, et al. Effect of a clinical practice guideline for pediatric complicated appendicitis. JAMA Surg. 2016;151(5):e160194. https://doi.org/10.1001/jamasurg.2016.0194.
66. Knott EM, Gasior AC, Ostlie DJ, Holcomb GW, St Peter SD. Decreased resource utilization since initiation of institutional clinical pathway for care of children with perforated appendicitis. J Pediatr Surg. 2013;48(6):1395–8. https://doi.org/10.1016/j.jpedsurg.2013.03.044.

Interventional Radiology as a Therapeutic Option for Complicated Appendicitis

9

Marcus Jarboe and Sara Smolinski-Zhao

Case Example

A 9-year-old previously healthy boy presented with right lower quadrant pain, WBC of 22 and an ultrasound (US) showing a 5.3 × 2 .2 cm thick-walled, complex fluid collection was identified in the pelvis (Fig. 9.1a). Magnetic resonance imaging (MRI) was performed, confirming a rim-enhancing fluid collection containing gas. A 12 French percutaneous drain was placed transrectally (Fig. 9.1b) with ultrasound guidance by interventional radiology (IR) on hospital day 1, with aspiration of 35 ml of purulent fluid.

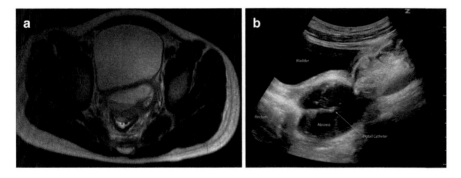

Fig. 9.1 (**a**) Axial T2W image of the pelvis showing an abscess anterior to the rectum. (**b**) Sagittal ultrasound image through the bladder showing transrectal drain in pelvic abscess

M. Jarboe (✉) · S. Smolinski-Zhao
Departments of Surgery and Vascular and Interventional Radiology, Mott Children's Hospital, University of Michigan, Ann Arbor, MI, USA
e-mail: marjarbo@med.umich.edu

© Springer Nature Switzerland AG 2019
C. J. Hunter (ed.), *Controversies in Pediatric Appendicitis*,
https://doi.org/10.1007/978-3-030-15006-8_9

Introduction

Acute appendicitis is one of the most common surgical pathologies in the United States, with perforation not uncommon in children and a reported 10–13% rate of associated abdominal abscess [1, 2]. Historically, the gold standard in treatment of abdominal abscesses has been with surgical drainage and debridement. Percutaneous drainage of an abdominal abscess was first reported in 1842 by a surgeon named Murray, who described the placement of a trocar and cannula into a liver collection "until adhesions formed between the liver and abdominal wall" [3]. Over the past several decades, however, percutaneous drainage (PD) has become the preferred method of treatment in adults and children alike as it is associated with a lower morbidity and mortality as compared to open surgical drainage [4–8]. PD is now recommended as first-line therapy for abscesses related to acute appendicitis by the World Society of Emergency Surgery and the Surgical Infection Society [9, 10].

Pre-procedure Evaluation

Abscess Identification

Acute appendicitis is a clinical diagnosis, though imaging has become a mainstay for complete evaluation. Classically, patients present with fever and abdominal pain, which over time localizes to the right lower quadrant. An abscess related to perforation may be identified on imaging, affecting patient management. Especially in small children, ultrasound is the preferred imaging modality as it avoids radiation exposure. Pediatric small body habitus lends itself well to identification of an enlarged appendix or a fluid collection by ultrasound. Diagnostic imaging findings of abscess are explained in more detail in an earlier chapter, but in general consist of thick-walled, often complex fluid collections. The appendix may also be identified in the region of the collection, with or without the offending appendicolith. If evaluation by ultrasound is limited and clinical suspicion remains high, MRI or CT may be considered. More recently, magnetic resonance imaging (MRI) is the preferred second-line imaging modality, as it avoids radiation exposure [11]. Abbreviated MRI protocols have been created to limit time on the scanner both to avoid sedation and conserve MRI time. For younger children, sedation still may be required for the use of MRI, the risk of which may be considered greater than the potential benefit. For this reason, CT is often the best second-line modality. A CT can be obtained in a manner of seconds, requiring no sedation or scheduling difficulties. Potential downsides of CT imaging include radiation exposure and protocols that may require oral contrast to better delineate bowel and appendix lumen. Transit of oral contrast may take up to 2–3 hours to reach the cecum.

Laboratory Studies

The most important preoperative laboratory studies are coagulation parameters, although evaluation may be deferred if the patient has no medical history of coagulation abnormality [12]. A platelet count greater than 50,000/uL is recommended by the Society of Interventional Radiology (SIR). An international normalized ratio (INR) less than 1.2, or less than 1.5 for urgent cases, is recommended [13]. A cutoff of 1.7 is used in many IR divisions. Occasionally, percutaneous drainage requires traversal of an organ, such as liver, stomach, or even bladder, which may be safely done, but more strongly requires evaluation of coagulation parameters due to the increased bleeding risk. Laboratory values outside of these recommendations require correction by pretreatment with oral vitamin K or fresh frozen plasma (FFP) for abnormal INR, cryoprecipitate, or platelet infusion. In many IR divisions, intra-procedural administration of FFP for an INR 1.7–2.0 and platelet transfusion for platelet counts of 25,000–50,000/uL are acceptable alternatives, which allow for timely patient care.

Antibiotic Therapy

Intravenous antibiotics are initiated at the time of patient diagnosis. If there is high concern for septicemia at the time of drain placement, coordinating the timing of the antibiotic to the 1 hour immediately prior to the procedure, or administering an additional dose, may be considered. Concern for septicemia is highest when the collection is present within a vascular organ, such as the liver [14].

Imaging Guidance for Drain Placement

Once an abscess is identified, the preferred method of management is by percutaneous drainage, which has lower morbidity and mortality risks than open drainage. US is largely the imaging modality of choice given its ability to provide real-time guidance and its radiation-free character. In adults or children with large body habitus, US visualization of the collection or adjacent structures may be limited. CT guidance provides for safe trajectory planning and procedural success. Small patient size makes US utilization more successful in children than in adults. When collections are present in the deep pelvis or encompassed by loops of bowel, however, US may not be safely performed, and CT is the preferred modality. Real-time MRI guidance is available at the author's institution and is used for core biopsies, but MRI-compatible guidewires and MRI-compatible drains are just now becoming available in the United States, and so MRI is not widely used at this time. Cone-beam CT with guidance abilities in IR suites which have the capable equipment and software. Cone-beam CT does produce radiation, however, and the image quality is somewhat less than a typical CT scan. The benefit of cone-beam CT is that it can provide real-time guidance.

Fig. 9.2 Laparoscopic ultrasound-assisted drainage of deep abscess in abdomen

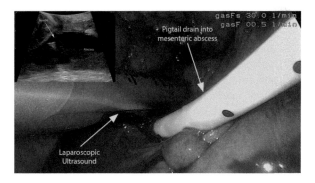

The real-time ability of US guidance has several advantages. The access needle and wire are visualized within the collection as they are placed. This allows for short procedure times, minimizing sedation requirements. The real-time guidance also provides a potential for greater control and accuracy of the path of the needle. CT-guided drain placement can take longer, as it is performed by instrument adjustment and stepping out of the procedure room for CT imaging. CT fluoroscopy may be utilized, if available, which can shorten the procedure. During CT fluoroscopy, 1–3 slice images are obtained by the use of a foot pedal. The interventionalist remains in the room or even with a hand on the instrument for guidance. Imaging is not truly real-time, but radiation dose is reduced by imaging smaller portions of the patient.

For deep pelvic collections, in close approximation to the rectum, transrectal drain placement may be considered. This allows for radiation avoidance by using a transrectal or transabdominal ultrasound probe for drain placement, detailed below.

For collections that are located more superiorly in the abdomen but covered by mesentery, or for those that are deep to multiple loops of bowel, laparoscopic-assisted ultrasound drainage of the abscess is effective. This allows easy manipulation of the bowel from the path of the drain (Fig. 9.2).

Indications for Percutaneous Drainage

Percutaneous drainage (PD) of peri-appendiceal abscess with interval appendectomy has been shown to have fewer complications than immediate appendectomy with a similar rate of clinical improvement [15–19]. Imaging findings to suggest infection include a thick wall around the collection, adjacent inflammation, wall enhancement, and the presence of air bubbles. Abscesses less than 3 cm are generally treated with antibiotic therapy alone, with a reported success rate of 88% based on an early study [20]. Aspiration can be performed if culture is desired for antibiotic tailoring. If a fistula is visualized during aspiration, a drain should be placed [21].

Contraindications to Percutaneous Drainage

PD of peri-appendiceal abscesses have been associated with a 4.5–26% failure rate in adults [7, 8]. A major contraindication to PD is inability to safely access the collection without injury to an adjacent organ, most importantly, a vascular structure

Fig. 9.3 Ultrasound-guided transhepatic placement of needle into a subphrenic abscess from perforated appendicitis for drain placement

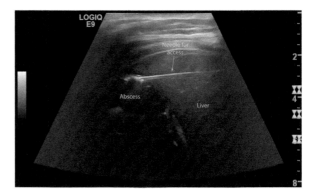

or bowel. Safe and effective transhepatic abscess drainage of upper abdominal collections has been described (Fig. 9.3), as has transvesicular drainage of pelvic fluid collections [16, 17]. Trans-pleural access should be avoided, to prevent spread of infection into the sterile pleural space. Bleeding diathesis or other coagulation abnormalities represent another important contraindication, though often risk of bleeding can be mitigated by transfusion of platelets or fresh frozen plasma to facilitate the less invasive PD placement and avoid open surgical intervention.

Procedural Considerations

The decision to place an abdominal drain is based on multidisciplinary discussion and consideration of patient-specific factors. After a discussion of the benefits, risks, and alternatives, informed consent is obtained from the patient's parent or legal guardian prior to the procedure. Sedation or general anesthesia is required for most pediatric drain placements, if not only to prevent patient discomfort but also to maximize the safety and success of the procedure by preventing patient movement. Liberal administration of local anesthetic is used to assist with pain management, paying particular attention to the peritoneal lining, which can be the most painful point of transgression. Attention should be paid to weight based maximum dosages to prevent systemic toxicity.

The choice of US or CT guidance is based on the location of the collection, the size of the patient, and the comfort level of the performing physician. When possible, ultrasound guidance is preferred, in accordance with ALARA principles (as low as reasonably achievable) [22, 23]. As discussed above, US is the preferred modality for procedural guidance, given the lack of ionizing radiation exposure and real-time guidance (Fig. 9.4). A potential downside in the use of US is that it cannot penetrate artifact related to bowel gas or gas within the collection itself. Careful comparison with prior imaging may provide reassurance that a gas-filled region on US represents the target collection, but typically then requires the use of another imaging modality to confirm catheter placement. This can be achieved either by CT to delineate the location of a guidewire, fluoroscopic imaging with contrast injection through the access needle, or cone-beam CT to prevent placement of a drain into bowel.

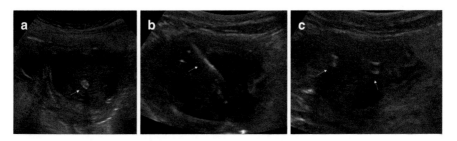

Fig. 9.4 (**a**) Sagittal grayscale Doppler ultrasonography demonstrates a complex fluid collection with internal echoes and a thick wall, consistent with abscess. An echogenic and shadowing focus in its central aspect represents an appendicolith (white arrow). (**b**) and (**c**) Transverse grayscale Doppler ultrasonography showing wire placement within the collection during drain placement (white arrow) and double echogenic lines of the catheter loop within the collection, with overall decrease in volume after aspiration

Basic Drainage Technique

There are two techniques utilized for drain placement: trocar technique and the more commonly used Seldinger technique. The trocar technique can be used when a collection is superficial or crosses a plane at high risk of loss of access during serial dilation. The Seldinger technique utilizes a smaller access needle and allows for confirmation of needle location within the collection prior to dilation and drain placement.

Regardless of the imaging modality utilized for guidance, preliminary imaging is performed to assess the safest route for drainage, avoiding vascular structures and abdominal organs. A radiopaque marking grid is placed in the expected region of safe access route based on prior imaging for CT-guided procedures. Patient comfort is also taken into account, placing the tube insertion site in a location that will not result in pressure on the tube while sitting or recumbent and avoiding a location which might be exposed to pressure related to clothing, if possible. When unavoidable, transgluteal route may be necessary, but can be associated with significant patient discomfort. For this reason, transrectal or transvaginal catheter placement is preferred for deep pelvic collections, located anterior to the rectum. Although placement can be slightly more challenging and there is a risk of catheter dislodgement, patient comfort is greater in these locations, and outcomes are similar.

Once a suitable access route is identified, sterile preparation of the access point is performed. For ultrasound-guided procedures, local anesthesia is then administered, and the access needle is advanced into the collection under direct visualization. Using the trocar method, the catheter itself with needle stylet is advanced through a small incision into the collection in one step. The catheter is advanced over the needle stylet, curling the distal "pigtail" loop within the collection. Aspiration then should yield fluid, and once confirmed within the collection, the loop is locked, catheter is secured to the skin by suture, and a dressing is placed.

Using Seldinger technique, either an 18-gauge needle or a 5French/19-gauge centesis catheter with introducer needle is advanced into the collection under ultrasound guidance. Aspiration yields fluid, confirming position within the collection, and the catheter is advanced over the needle into the collection further. The needle is exchanged for a guidewire, over which the centesis catheter is exchanged for the drainage catheter after serial tract dilation, if necessary. The trocar method may be preferred for transrectal or transvaginal drainage, as serial dilation of the tract may dislodge the guiding wire from the collection during exchanges.

When using ultrasound for transrectal or transvaginal guidance, a curved (for larger children) or linear (for small children) probe may be used for visualization of the pelvic collection from the anterior abdomen, taking advantage of the phenomenon of acoustic enhancement through the bladder for visualization of the collection and needle (Fig. 9.1a). Acoustic enhancement consists of the characteristic of simple fluid (urine, in this case) to appear to delineate deeper structures with more clarity and echogenicity (brightness), as soundwaves are attenuated less by the fluid than by adjacent soft tissue structures. Using the trocar technique, the drain with blunt stylet is then advanced through the rectum with a finger near its tip toward the collection. The blunt stylet is then exchanged for the needle stylet and advanced through rectal/vaginal wall into the collection under direct visualization. Alternatively, an 18-gauge needle can be advanced through the rectum in a similar manner, using a plastic tubing which has been split longitudinally for a modified peel-away sheath to protect the rectal/vaginal wall from injury during needle advancement. If the patient is too large, however, the transabdominal technique will not be successful. A rectal/vaginal ultrasound probe is then used, with or without the needle guide attachment, to place the needle into the collection alongside to the probe. The catheter is then secured to the inner thigh using an adhesive catheter securement device.

A similar technique is employed for CT guidance. A radiopaque grid is used to mark the optimal insertion site, and a trajectory is mapped out on imaging. The depth of the collection from the skin surface is measured, and after sterile preparation, local anesthetic is administered, and the anesthetic needle is advanced through the skin at the determined angle to access the site. Repeat imaging is performed, either using a foot pedal for CT fluoroscopy or with 5–7 axial slices centered on the needle insertion site. Once a satisfactory trajectory is confirmed using the small anesthetic needle, an incision is made, and an 18-gauge needle or 5French/19-gauge centesis catheter. The introducer needle is then advanced to determine the depth at the appropriate angle. Aspiration can then be performed, and if fluid is aspirated, a guidewire is advanced through the needle or centesis catheter after removal of its introducer needle. Repeat imaging may be performed to confirm wire location within the collection, or serial tract dilation with catheter placement is performed without repeat imaging if there is confidence in wire location. Once the catheter is advanced into the collection, aspiration should yield additional fluid, the loop is locked, and final CT imaging is performed to document/assess catheter position. The catheter is then secured to the skin with suture and a dressing applied.

Regardless of technique, the catheter is attached to closed suction drainage bulb (e.g., a Jackson-Pratt) or a drainage bag for gravity drainage. JP bulb use may be preferred, given the likely superior drainage of thick pus by suction.

Post-procedure Management

Patients should be assessed daily for persistent/recurrent fever or worsening abdominal pain. Drain output should be recorded for every 8–12 hour shift by nursing staff. 5–10 ml saline flushes every 8–12–24 hours is recommended to prevent catheter occlusion by debris [1, 24, 25]. The volume of the flush is subtracted from the total output volume at the time of output documentation.

Catheter removal is considered when the patient has remained afebrile, is clinically improving, and catheter output is less than 5–10 ml over 24 hours [26–28]. No follow-up imaging is required if the patient has clinically improved and total output is as expected for the size and complexity of the collection. Repeat imaging is performed if drain output is lower than expected, the collection is complex, or output abruptly decreases and there is concern for catheter clogging. The presence of persistent fever or lack of clinical improvement recommends repeat imaging to assess for residual fluid or a new collection [24]. The body can wall off the drain from the rest of the abscess, or the complexity of the abscess can preclude complete drainage. In these instances manipulation of the drain to lyse adhesions or placement of a second drain can be considered. Use of persistent drain output prompts repeat imaging to assess for fistulae to bowel, which may include a tube sinogram under fluoroscopy.

Complications

Complications of PD may take place at the time of the procedure or in a delayed manner, as a result of catheter presence. Severe complications occur most commonly at the time of drain placement and include a drug-related allergic reaction or cardiac arrest/respiratory failure due to oversedation. Spread of infection to adjacent compartments or organs may occur as a delayed complication, particularly if care is not taken to avoid crossing the pleural space, for example. During transhepatic abscess drainage, careful evaluation under fluoroscopy for fistula formation to bile ducts or vascular structures is important prior to drain removal [16]. Minor complications include catheter kinking, obstruction, or dislodgement after placement. Catheter replacement depends on the clinical status of the patient and the presence of residual collection.

Bleeding is a risk of variable magnitude which depends on the location of the abscess. Abscesses within or adjacent to vascular organs, such as liver or spleen, carry a higher risk of bleeding. Proximity to vascular structures in the pelvis may increase the risk of bleeding during catheter placement. In the setting of venous injury, catheter upsize or temporary capping of the drain serves to tamponade the bleed and typically results in resolution. Persistent or pulsatile bleeding is suggestive of an arterial injury, which is assessed by CT angiography and treated by fluoroscopic angiography with embolization of the bleeding vessel. Large vessel laceration requires urgent surgical management.

Transient bacteremia has been reported in up to 5% of cases, likely related to hypervascularity in the wall of the abscess [29]. When multiple fluid collections are present and there is question as to the potential sterility of one or more, it is important to use new sterile materials for accessing and draining each collection to avoid spread of infection from one to the other [30]. Local skin infections can occur if a drainage catheter is present for a prolonged period of time. Treatment may either be with antibiotic therapy or placement of a new drain away from the infected incision.

Malposition of the catheter during placement is another risk and most commonly involves the placement of a drain into bowel. This may be immediately recognized at the time of the procedure or may be identified after persistent drain output is noted. Diagnosis may be by repeat imaging or by fluoroscopic tube evaluation. Management of an abscess drain in the bowel is either by surgical repair or delayed catheter removal after tract maturation.

Conclusion

Percutaneous drainage of abdominal abscesses has become a frequently used and valuable alternative to open surgical intervention, with similar outcomes in clinical improvement and lower morbidity and mortality. With appropriate consideration for potential risks, the procedure can be performed in conjunction with interval appendectomy to optimize outcomes in this patient population.

Clinical Pearls

- Coagulation studies are not routinely needed prior to percutaneous drainage.
- MRI and US can be used to evaluate postoperative abscess collections instead of CT avoiding unnecessary ionizing radiation.
- Transrectal abscess drainage in the deep pelvis is often better tolerated than transgluteal drains.

References

1. Hogan MJ. Appendiceal abscess drainage. Tech Vasc Interv Radiol. 2003;6(4):205–14.
2. Whyte C, Levin T, Harris BH. Early decisions in perforated appendicitis in children: lessons from a study of nonoperative management. J Pediatr Surg. 2008;43(8):1459–63.
3. Briddon CK III. Surgical observations in the treatment of the diseases and accidents of the liver. Ann Surg. 1885;2(7):51–61.
4. Towbin RB. Pediatric interventional procedures in the 1980s: a period of development, growth, and acceptance. Radiology. 1989;170(3 Pt 2):1081–90.

5. Mueller PR. The evolution of image-guided percutaneous abscess drainage: a short history. Semin Interv Radiol. 2003;20(3):171–6.
6. Brolin RE, Nosher JL, Leiman S, et al. Percutaneous catheter versus open surgical drainage in the treatment of abdominal abscesses. Am Surg. 1984;50(2):102–8.
7. Andersson RE, Petzold MG. Nonsurgical treatment of appendiceal abscess or phlegmon: a systematic review and meta-analysis. Ann Surg. 2007;246:741–8.
8. Maxfield MW, Schuster KM, Bokhari J, et al. Predictive factors for failure of nonoperative management in perforated appendicitis. J Trauma Acute Care Surg. 2014;76:976–81.
9. DiSaverio S, Birindelli A, Kelly MD, et al. WSES Jerusalem guidelines for diagnosis and treatment of acute appendicitis. World J Emerg Surg. 2016;11:34.
10. Mazuski JE, Tessier JM, May AK, et al. The Surgical Infection Society revised guidelines on the management of intra-abdominal infection. Surg Infect. 2017;18:1–76.
11. Dillman JR, Gadepalli S, Sroufe NS, et al. Equivocal pediatrix appendicitis: unenhanced MR imaging protocol for nonsedated children- a clinical effectiveness study. Radiology. 2016;279(1):216–25.
12. Brown C, Kang L, Kim ST. Percutaneous drainage of abdominal and pelvic abscesses in children. Semin Interv Radiol. 2012;29:286–94.
13. Hogan MJ, Marshalleck FE, Sidhu MK, et al. Quality improvement guidelines for pediatric abscess and fluid drainage. J Vasc Interv Radiol. 2012;23:1397–402.
14. Thomas J, Turner SR, Nelson RC, Paulson EK. Postprocedure sepsis in imaging-guided percutaneous hepatic abscess drainage: how often does it occur? Am J Roentgenol. 2006;186(5):1419–22.
15. Shuler FW, Newman CN, Angood PB, et al. Nonoperative management for intra-abdominal abscesses. Am Surg. 1996;62:218–22.
16. Ciftci TT, Akinci D, Akhan O. Percutaneous transhepatic drainage of inaccessible postoperative abdominal abscesses. AJR Am J Roentgenol. 2012 Feb;198(2):477–81.
17. Ayyagari RR, Yeh C, Arici M, et al. Image-guided transvesicular drainage of pelvic fluid collections: a safe and effective alternative approach. J Vasc Interv Radiol. 2016;27(5):689–93.
18. Oliak D, Yamini D, Vm U, et al. Initial nonoperative management for periappendiceal abscess. Dis Colon Rectum. 2001;44:936–41.
19. Simillis C, Symeonides P, Shorthouse AJ, Tekkis PP. A meta-analysis comparing conservative treatment versus acute appendectomy for complicated appendicitis (abscess or phlegmon). Surgery. 2010;147:818–29.
20. Jeffrey RB, Federle MP, Tolentino CS. Periappendiceal inflammatory masses: CT-directed management and clinical outcome in 70 patients. Radiology. 1988;167(1):13–6.
21. Kerlan RK Jr, Jeffrey RB Jr, Pogany AC, Ring EJ. Abdominal abscesses with low-output fistula: successful percutaneous drainage. Radiology. 1985;155(1):73–5.
22. Krishnamoorthi R, Ramarajan N, Wang NE, et al. Effectiveness of a staged US and CT protocol for the diagnosis of pediatric appendicitis: reducing radiation exposure in the age of ALARA. Radiology. 2011;259(1):231–9.
23. Strauss K, Kaste SC. The ALARA (as low as reasonably achievable) concept in pediatric interventional and fluoroscopic imaging: striving to keep radiation doses as low as possible during fluoroscopy of pediatric patients – a white paper executive summary. Radiology. 2006;240(3):621–2.
24. Gervais DA, Brown SD, Connolly SA, et al. Percutaneous imaging-guided abdominal and pelvic abscess drainage in children. Radiographics. 2004;24(3):737–54.
25. Beland MD, Da G, Hahn PF, et al. CT-guided transgluteal drainage of deep pelvic abscesses: indicates, technique, procedure-related complications, and clinical outcome. Radiographics. 2002;22(6):1353–67.
26. Rajak CL, Gupta S, Jain S, et al. Percutaneous treatment of liver abscesses: needle aspiration versus catheter drainage. AJR Am J Roentgenol. 1998;170(4):1035–9.
27. Hogan MJ, Hoffer FA. Biopsy and drainage techniques in children. Tech Vasc Interv Radiol. 2010;13(4):206–13.
28. vanSonnenberg E, Ferrucci JT Jr, Mueller PR, et al. Percutaneous drainage of abscesses and fluid collections: technique, results and applications. Radiology. 1982;142(1):1–10.

29. Lorenz J, Thomas JL. Complications of percutaneous fluid drainage. Semin Interv Radiol. 2006;23:194–204.
30. Heneghan JP, Everts RJ, Nelson RC. Multiple fluid collections: CT- or US-guided aspiration-evaluation of microbiologic results and implications for clinical practice. Radiology. 1999;212:669–72.

Timing of Appendectomy for Acute Appendicitis: Can Surgery Wait?

Shawn J. Rangel

Case Example
A 9-year-old boy presents at 10 PM with right lower quadrant abdominal pain and undergoes an ultrasound confirming appendicitis. The on-call surgeon prefers to perform the appendectomy immediately with concern that delay may lead to perforation. The anesthesiologist on call challenges the need for immediate surgery and remarks that the cost of bringing in an operative team in the middle of the night is not justified from either a fiscal or "standard of care" perspective. After further debate, they agree to book the case for 6:30 AM the following morning before electively scheduled cases begin.

Introduction

The scenario described above is likely to be quite common; controversy and lack of consensus around the safety and fiscal implications of delaying appendectomy until the following morning exist even among pediatric surgeons. The published literature would suggest a growing trend toward acceptance of operative delay (at least until the following day for patients presenting the night before), but is this justified by the available evidence? What is the impact of time to appendectomy (TTA) following hospital presentation on the risk of appendiceal perforation and postoperative complications? How does delay of appendectomy impact resource

S. J. Rangel (✉)
Department of Pediatric and Thoracic Surgery, Boston Children's Hospital, Boston, MA, USA

Harvard Medical School, Boston, MA, USA
e-mail: Shawn.Rangel@childrens.harvard.edu

© Springer Nature Switzerland AG 2019
C. J. Hunter (ed.), *Controversies in Pediatric Appendicitis*,
https://doi.org/10.1007/978-3-030-15006-8_10

utilization and hospital cost? Several studies have attempted to shed light on these questions using a wide variety of analytic methods, some with conflicting results. The goal of this review was to provide a critical review of the available literature to shed light on the influence of treatment delay on both clinical and fiscal outcomes. Specifically, we wished to explore this relationship in the context of three categories: (1) risk of complicated or perforated appendicitis found at operative exploration, (2) risk of adverse events in the postoperative period, and (3) resource utilization, including hospital cost, length of hospital stay, and readmission.

Literature Review

Literature searches were performed in English using Medline, PubMed, and pertinent Cochrane reviews. A comprehensive literature search was conducted using the following search terms: appendicitis, appendectomy, timeliness, delay, timing of surgery, perforation, and complicated appendicitis. All identified studies were manually reviewed for outcomes of interest rather than using additional search terms to be comprehensive. Further cross-checking was performed by reviewing the reference list associated with all studies included in the reference list of this review.

For the purpose of this review, only studies exclusively reporting on outcomes in patients 18 years of age and younger were included. This decision was based on the evidence-based premise that "children are not small adults" with respect to factors that may impact the measurable association between treatment delay and outcomes. These include factors influencing timelines of presentation, disease progression, and rate of perforation at hospital presentation. Furthermore, it was the opinion of the author that the current pool of pediatric evidence was of sufficient volume and rigor to stand alone without the need to include adult-specific data (which could compromise both generalizability and external validity).

Studies that reported outcomes associated with treatment delay in calendar days rather than hours were also excluded. This was done to focus the review on studies that were calibrated to address the contemporary clinical question as to whether a modest delay in appendectomy (i.e., the next morning for a patient presenting in the evening the night before) is a safe and fiscally reasonable practice. Studies reporting outcomes in calendar days (large database studies such as KID and NIS) are likely to misclassify many patients when attempting to address this clinical question. To illustrate further, a patient who presents at 11:30 PM and then undergoes an appendectomy 2 hours later at 1:30 AM the next calendar day would be categorized as a "next day" (2 calendar days) appendectomy, while a patient who presents at 12:30 AM and then undergoes appendectomy 20 hours later at 8:30 PM would be considered a "same day" (1 calendar day) appendectomy. Such misclassification will bias the analysis toward the null hypothesis (no difference between same day and next day appendectomy) even if an increased risk of adverse outcomes actually exists.

Discussion

Treatment Delay and Risk of Perforated Disease

Nine studies were identified that explored an association between timing of appendectomy and risk of complicated or perforated appendicitis. Collectively, these studies included 8473 patients from 42 different hospitals. Seven (78%) of studies were retrospective and five (56%) were single-center experiences (Table 10.1).

Overall, seven (78%) of the nine studies did not find an association between delay and risk of perforation or complicated appendicitis. However, it should be noted that the available literature pool was quite heterogeneous with respect to analytic methods and definitions for both exposures and outcomes. These included a lack of standardized definitions for assessing perforation and complicated disease, as well as differences between studies in measuring time from presentation or admission to appendectomy. A formal meta-analysis to aggregate data across studies was therefore not possible.

Given the heterogeneity of available data, a critical review of the potential sources of bias associated with different study designs and analytic methods is important to gauge the strength of different studies. In this regard, two studies in the review were identified as prospective cohort designs. Based on the relatively well-documented and objective nature of ED presentation and surgical start time (exposure components), prospective study designs are not likely to provide more accurate TTA estimates compared to their retrospective counterparts. Furthermore, none of these studies specifically indicated how their prospective methodology improved the capture and accuracy of outcomes data (status of perforation or complicated appendicitis) from pathology and operative reports. Given these considerations, prospective studies should not be considered superior in their validity to retrospective study designs in this review.

The influence of clinical disease severity on timing of appendectomy is a potentially important source of bias and one that may greatly vary across hospitals. It is well established that most perforations in children occur prior to hospital presentation, and patients who are perforated on presentation typically have more severe clinical presentations compared to those who are not. Some hospitals may treat children with more severe presentations more expeditiously, while others may elect to obtain additional cross-sectional imaging or proceed with a period of resuscitation prior to appendectomy. Depending on a hospital's diagnostic and treatment approach, children who are perforated at time of presentation may have different TTA profiles at baseline compared to those who are not. This effect could bias the analyses between TTA and perforated disease in either direction. Early operative management of children with a pre-existing perforation would bias the analysis away from an association between TTA and perforation (even if one actually exists), while delayed operative intervention for pre-existing perforations may bias the analyses toward an association (even if one didn't exist). The former effect (early management of more severe disease) may explain why some studies have demonstrated a trend toward lower perforation rates with longer TTA (e.g., a "protective" effect with delay) [1].

Table 10.1 Summary of published studies reporting the association between timing of appendectomy and outcomes in the pediatric age group

Citations	Study timeline (N)	Study design	Analytic method/ exposure groups	Outcomes definitions/criteria	Outcomes associated with delay (main results)		
					Perforation	Adverse events	Resource utilization
Serres et al. [11]	2012–2014 (2116)	Multicenter retrospective cohort (16 hospitals)	Multivariable regression (exposure analyzed in quartiles of TTA)	Standardized cost (each billed item recalculated using the median cost from all 16 hospitals)	N/A	N/A	*Increased resource utilization found*; the longest quartile of TTA was associated with 23% higher total cost ($1589/case, RR:1.23, 95%CI:1.14–1.32, $p < 0.001$) and 53% higher room-associated cost ($906/case,RR:1.53, 95%CI:1.35–1.74, $p < 0.001$) compared to the shortest quartile
Serres et al. [10]	2012–2014 (2429)	Multicenter retrospective cohort (23 hospitals)	Multivariable regression (exposure analyzed in 1 hour increments); rates of complicated appendicitis also examined at each hospital (before/after their respective median TTAs)	Standardized NSQIP-Pediatric criteria used for complicated appendicitis (operative reports reviewed for free fecalith, abscess, diffuse fibropurulent exudate, visible hole) and all adverse event outcomes	*No increased risk found*; OR: 0.99 (95%CI:0.97–1.02) for each hour of delay in pooled analysis; no increased risk found for 22 of 23 hospitals when examined individually	*No increased risk found*; for each hour delay: SSI OR: 0.96 (95%CI:0.88–1.04), OSI OR: 1.00 (95%CI:0.95–1.05), drainage procedures OR: 1.02 (95%CI:0.97–1.07), unplanned reoperation OR: 1.00 (95%CI:0.93–1.07)	*No increased risk for readmissions*; OR: 1.01 (95%CI:0.99–1.04) for each hour of delay; *increased LOS found*: 0.06 days of increased LOS for each hour of treatment delay (95%CI:0.03–0.08 days)

| Stevenson et al. [4] | Not reported (955) | Multicenter retrospective cohort (10 hospitals) | Multivariable regression (exposure analyzed in 1 hour increments) | Review of operative reports using standardized criteria for complicated appendicitis developed by study consortium (operative reports reviewed for perforation, rupture, complex appendicitis, purulent material, abscess) | *No increased risk found;* OR for all patients: 1.00 (95%CI:0.96–1.05) for each hour of delay, OR for subgroup analyses of longer delays between 12 and 24 hours, 0.93 (95%CI:0.79–1.08) for each hour of delay | N/A | N/A |
| Almstrom et al. [1] | 2006–2013 (2756) | Single-center retrospective cohort | Multivariable regression (exposures groups: <12 vs. 12–24 hours) | Pathology and operative reports (operative reports reviewed for visible hole, purulent peritonitis, abscess) | *No increased risk found;* OR for delayed group: 0.79 (95%CI:0.87–1.36) | *No increased risk found;* SSI OR: 0.69 (95%CI:0.35–1.36), OSI OR: 0.76 (95%CI:0.48–1.20), reoperation OR: 1.13 (95%CI:0.41–3.16) | *No increased utilization found;* readmission OR: 0.79 (95%CI:0.49–1.26) |

(continued)

Table 10.1 (continued)

Citations	Study timeline (N)	Study design	Analytic method/ exposure groups	Outcomes definitions/criteria	Outcomes associated with delay (main results)		
					Perforation	Adverse events	Resource utilization
Boomer et al. [9]	2010–2012 (1388)	Multicenter retrospective cohort (6 hospitals)	Multivariable regression and Cochran-Armitage test for trend using SSI as outcome. Complicated and uncomplicated appendicitis identified from operative reports and used for risk stratification, not for outcomes (exposures groups: <4 vs. 4–8 vs. 8–12 vs. 12–16 vs. >16 hours)	Standardized NSQIP-Pediatric criteria used for SSI outcomes; chart review used to categorize simple and complicated appendicitis for risk stratification	*No increased risk found; regression p-value for delayed groups as both categorical and continuous variable >0.1 for both simple and complicated subgroups (no additional data provided)*	*No increased risk found*; time not identified in multivariable regression as significant (OR data not provided in manuscript), SSI rates (<4 hours): 0.0 vs. >16 hours): 0.0 vs. 0.9% ($p = 0.58$) for simple appendicitis, 5.0 vs. 4.0% ($p = 1.0$) for complicated appendicitis	N/A
Meltzer et al. [3]	1998–2014 (857)	Multicenter retrospective cohort (5 hospitals)	Multivariable regression (exposures groups: <3 vs. 3–6 vs. >6 hours)	Operative reports (no further detail provided)	*Increased risk found*; OR for delayed group: 1.02 (95%CI:1.00–1.04) for each hour of delay	N/A	N/A

Gurien et al. [13]	2009–2012 (484)	Single-center retrospective cohort	Multivariable regression for perforation (exposure group: <16 vs. >16 hours); chi-square tests for adverse event analyses	*No increased risk found; OR for delayed group: 1.0 (95%CI:0.96–1.04)*	*No increased risk found;* SSI OR: 0.69 (95%CI:0.35–1.36), OSI OR: 0.76 (95%CI:0.48–1.20). reoperation OR: 1.13 (95%CI:0.41–3.16)	N/A
Manderville et al. [14]	2002–2010 (230)	Single-center prospective cohort	Multivariable regression (exposures groups: <3 vs. 3–6 vs. >6 hours)	*No increased risk found; OR for delayed groups:* 0.81 (95%CI:0.35–1.88) for 4–6 hour group, 0.98 (95%CI:0.48–1.96)	N/A	*No increased utilization found*; no difference in median LOS or operative time found across groups
Bonadio et al. [2]	2004–2010 (248)	Single-center retrospective cohort	Multivariable regression (exposure groups: <8 vs. 8–16 vs. >16 hours)	*Increased risk found; OR for* delayed group: 2.05 (95%CI:1.00–3.10) for 8–16 hours, 4.22 (95%CI:3.17–5.27) for >16 hours; OR for all patients: 1.10 (95%CI:1.04–1.16) for each hour of delay	N/A	N/A

Pathology reports; perforated appendicitis as diagnosed by preoperative imaging excluded

Pathology and operative reports (no further detail provided)

Pathology and operative reports (operative reports reviewed for "diagnosis of perforation")

(continued)

Table 10.1 (continued)

Citations	Study timeline (N)	Study design	Analytic method/ exposure groups	Outcomes definitions/criteria	Outcomes associated with delay (main results)		
					Perforation	Adverse events	Resource utilization
Boomer et al. [12]	2010–2012 (1338)	Single-center retrospective cohort	Multivariable regression and Cochran-Armitage test for trend using SSI as outcome. Complicated and uncomplicated appendicitis identified from operative reports and used for risk stratification, not for outcomes (exposures groups: <4 vs. 4–8 vs. 8–12 vs. 12–16 vs. >16 hours)	Operative reports (to categorize simple and complicated appendicitis for risk stratification)	N/A	*No increased risk found*; time not identified in multivariable regression as significant (OR data not provided in manuscript), SSI rates (<4 hours vs. >16 hours): 2.4 vs. 1.5% (p = 0.44) for simple appendicitis, 11.1 vs. 15.2% (p = 0.44) for complicated appendicitis	N/A
Yardeni et al. [15]	1998–2001 (126)	Single-center retrospective cohort	Multivariable regression (exposures groups: <6 vs. 6–12 vs. >12 hours); chi-square tests used to compare proportions across groups for adverse events	Pathology reports (no further detail provided)	*No increased risk found*; regression p-value for delayed groups = 0.37 (no other data provided)	*No increased risk found*; OSI/drainage rates (<6 hours vs. >6 hours): 2.6 vs. 5.7% (p = 0.067), OSI/drainage rates (<6 hours vs. >6 hours): 2.6 vs. 5.7% (p = 0.067),	*Trend in increased utilization found for LOS; <6 hours (1.7 days) vs. >6 hours (2.5 days), p = 0.06; increased utilization found for median cost; <6 hours ($7366) vs. >12 hours ($9893), p = 0.02*

TTA time to appendectomy, *SSI* surgical site infection, *OSI* organ space infection, *LOS* length of stay, *OR* odds ratio, *CI* confidence interval

In an attempt to mitigate bias associated with unknown perforation status on presentation, several studies have reported using computed tomography (CT) to exclude patients with perforation suspected on imaging [2–4]. However, the lack of sensitivity for differentiating complicated from uncomplicated disease using cross-sectional imaging has been well documented in both the radiology and surgical literature [5–7]. Computed tomography may be quite sensitive for diagnosing late presentations with rim-enhancing fluid collections, although the far more common scenario is early perforation with a non-enhancing adjacent fluid collection and localized fat stranding. Gangrenous appendicitis without perforation is frequently encountered in these cases, and often times the radiology read is equivocal. Furthermore, the generalizability of results from these studies may be limited as patients undergoing CT scans are arguably a different cohort than those that undergo ultrasound only.

Many different approaches have been used for identifying and defining outcomes (perforated and complicated appendicitis). Use of histology alone can both over- and underestimate perforation rates depending on operative and pathology factors. Overestimation can occur from holes made in a gangrenous appendix during its removal, while underestimation may occur if only a small portion of the appendix is sectioned to confirm the diagnosis of appendicitis during pathology evaluation. Review of operative reports has been proposed as a more clinically relevant means to establish the presence of both perforation and complicated disease. In this regard, histological perforation has poorly defined correlates for adverse events and increased resource utilization, while the presence of certain intraoperative findings (e.g., abscess and extraluminal fecaliths) has well established associations with clinically relevant consequences (e.g., organ space infections and increased hospital cost) [8]. However, details regarding the criteria used to identify complicated appendicitis from operative reports were often poorly described and not standardized in most studies, with only four studies (all multicenter study designs) specifically describing efforts in their methodology to standardize and audit for the purpose of quality assurance [4, 9–11].

When considering the many different sources of potential bias described above, we would caution that the generalizability and external validity of any single-center experience may be greatly limited. A multicenter study design to balance out variation in disease severity-associated treatment delay coupled with a standardized methodology for assessing outcomes would provide the best possible analyses. Four studies included in this review included multicenter analyses, although two deserve special mention given their particularly wide scope and rigorous study designs. The first was a multicenter study of 955 patients from 10 hospitals which was sponsored by the Pediatric Emergency Medicine Collaborative Research Committee of the American Academy of Pediatrics [4]. The investigators used a broad definition of appendiceal perforation which included both the presence of a physical hole and indirect findings of perforation (e.g., abscess). Case definitions were defined a priori in a written manual of operations, and site investigators received detailed instruction on interpreting and coding of radiologic, operative, and pathology reports. Data quality checks were performed monthly with discrepant findings reviewed and corrected for the purpose of quality assurance. Following regression analyses adjusting for a wide variety of patient-level factors, the investigators found no increase in the risk of perforated appendicitis with increasing time from ED presentation to appendectomy. Furthermore, no association between TTA and perforated appendicitis was found in subgroup analyses of patients who were believed to be non-perforated based on CT obtained in the ED.

The second study included 2429 children undergoing appendectomy at 23 hospitals as part of a national collaborative supported by the American College of Surgeon's National Surgical Quality Improvement Program-Pediatric (NSQIP-Pediatric) [10]. The investigators utilized a definition for complicated disease that was developed and standardized through NSQIP's Data Definitions Committee and based on criteria associated with adverse outcomes and resource utilization. A standardized manual of operations and instructional webinar was created for study participants, and a clinical support network was established to ensure data collection integrity. Following regression analyses adjusting for a wide variety of patient-level factors, the investigators found no increase in the risk of complicated appendicitis with increasing time from ED presentation to appendectomy. It is notable that the results of this regression analysis using TTA as a continuous variable were remarkably similar to that from the emergency medicine collaborative study (OR for each hour of treatment delay: 1.00 [95%CI:0.96–1.05] vs. 0.99 [95%CI:0.97–1.02]). The investigators also performed a secondary analysis at the hospital level for each of the 23 participating hospitals. Comparison groups (early and late TTA) were defined by each hospital's median TTA. Exposures were defined in this manner to compare rates of complicated disease within a timeframe sensitive to each hospital infrastructure and diagnostic practices and to provide insight into whether a hospital could potentially reduce its rate of complicated disease by "shifting" patients from its late group to its early group. An increased risk of complicated appendicitis was found at only 1 of the 23 hospitals examined (Fig. 10.1). This finding suggests that internal efforts on behalf of individual hospitals to decrease their TTA (e.g., to improve the efficiency of the diagnostic process) would likely not lead to a reduction in their rate of complicated disease.

Treatment Delay and Risk of Adverse Events

Six studies reported outcomes associated with adverse events in the postoperative period. Several different types of adverse events were reported including surgical site infections (SSI), organ space infections (OSI), small bowel obstruction, percutaneous drainage procedures, and reoperation. Two studies used standardized NSQIP criteria for adverse event outcomes, while the remainder provided little detail around both definitions and efforts to standardize data collection and definitions. Issues surrounding heterogeneity of definitions and analytic bias were similar to that described above for perforation; however, it is noteworthy that none of the six studies examining adverse events found an association with treatment delay. These

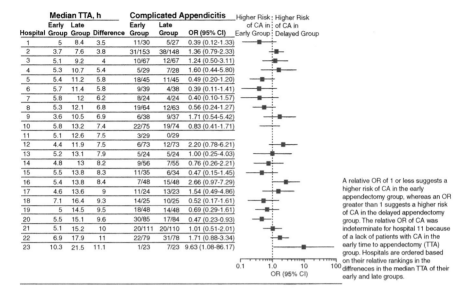

Fig. 10.1 Risk of complicated appendicitis associated with treatment delay at 23 children's hospitals. Hospitals are ordered from top to bottom by median time to appendectomy (TTA), and comparison groups (early and late TTA) were defined by each hospital's median TTA. Exposures were defined in this manner to compare rates of complicated disease within a timeframe sensitive to each hospital infrastructure and diagnostic practices and to provide insight into whether a hospital could potentially reduce its rate of complicated disease by decreasing its TTA relative to its median TTA. (Reproduced with permission from Serres et al. [10], Copyright© (2017) American Medical Association. All rights reserved)

included the two rigorous multicenter studies described above which also examined adverse event rates in addition to rates of complicated appendicitis [9, 10].

Treatment Delay and Impact on Resource Utilization

Five studies examined the association between treatment delay and resource utilization, including three reporting length of stay (LOS), two reporting readmission rates, and two reporting hospital cost. Two of the single-center studies examining LOS found either no association with treatment delay or a trend toward increased LOS. However, the number of patients included in these studies was relatively small which may have led to underpowered analyses. In a rigorously designed multicenter study of 2116 patients from 16 children's hospitals, Serres et al. found a 0.06-day increase in LOS associated with each hour of treatment delay [11]. Both studies examining hospital cost found an association with increased treatment delay, and these included the same study by Serres et al. which found a 23% difference in hospital cost between the longest and shortest quartiles of TTA (Table 10.2) [11]. None of the studies examining readmission rates found an association with readmission.

Table 10.2 Influence of time to appendectomy (categorized by hospital-specific quartiles) on hospital cost in 2116 patients at 16 children's hospitals

	Time to appendectomy				
	1st quartile	2nd quartile	3rd quartile	4th quartile	
Overall costs					
Adjusted mean	$6967	$7682	$7798	$8556	<0.001
Rate ratio (95% confidence intervals)	Ref	1.10 (1.03–1.18)	1.12 (1.04–1.2)	1.23 (1.14–1.32)	
Operating room costs					
Adjusted mean	$3739	$3930	$4084	$4005	<0.001
Rate ratio (95% confidence intervals)	Ref	1.05 (1.01–1.09)	1.09 (1.05–1.14)	1.07 (1.03–1.12)	
Operating room time-based costs					
Adjusted mean	$1400	$1360	$1370	$1332	0.22
Rate ratio (95% confidence intervals)	Ref	0.97 (093, 1.02)	0.98 (0.93, 1.03)	0.95 (0.91, 1.00)	
Operating room fixed costs					
Adjusted mean	$1912	$2188	$2266	$2305	<0.001
Rate ratio (95% confidence intervals)	Ref	1.14 (1.09, 1.2)	1.18 (1.12, 1.25)	1.21 (1.14, 1.27)	
Room costs					
Adjusted mean	$1695	$1723	$1853	$2601	<0.001
Rate ratio (95% confidence intervals)	Ref	1.01 (0.9–1.15)	1.09 (097–1.24)	1.53 (1.35–1.74)	

Reprinted from Serres et al. [11], with permission from Elsevier

Conclusion

Based on currently available data in the pediatric literature, we conclude there is compelling evidence to support the premise that a modest delay in appendectomy (e.g., the next calendar day for children presenting the night before) is a safe and reasonable practice. Although two studies (including one multicenter study) did show an increased risk of perforation with treatment delay, it is important to emphasize that none of the studies in this review demonstrated an increased risk for adverse events associated with measurable patient harm.

Although the data would suggest that treatment delay does not increase the risk of clinically relevant adverse outcomes within the first 24 hours, it is important to note that the influence of timely antibiotic administration was not addressed in many of the included studies. The role of antibiotics in arresting the progression of appendicitis has been well established in studies where antibiotics have been used as primary (and definitive) treatment for early appendicitis. It is plausible that antibiotics may also have played a role in mitigating the risk of perforation for the studies included in this review. Timely administration of antibiotics immediately following diagnosis should therefore be considered an essential part of any management strategy.

Finally, the relationship between TTA and resource utilization is complex and dependent on the outcomes examined. Longer TTA does not appear to be associated with hospital readmission, but does appear to be associated with increased cost and LOS, particularly in larger studies that include multiple hospitals with longer median TTAs. These results are perhaps not surprising; readmission encounters are often associated with adverse events such as organ space infections (of which there was no association with treatment delay), while longer delays to definitive treatment for any condition will likely lead to longer time in the hospital with increased charges associated with bed days and nursing shifts, among others. The ultimate decision surrounding timing of appendectomy in any hospital should balance the benefits of a timely intervention against the hospital's available resources.

Clinical Pearls

- A modest delay in appendectomy is acceptable; however antibiotics should be initiated in a timely fashion.
- Delay in appendectomy does not appear to significantly increase complications.
- Longer TTA is not associated with a higher readmission rate, but does correlate with an increased cost and length of stay.

References

1. Almstrom M, Svensson JF, Patkova B, Svenningsson A, Wester T. In-hospital surgical delay does not increase the risk for perforated appendicitis in children: a single-center retrospective cohort study. Ann Surg. 2017;265(3):616–21. https://doi.org/10.1097/SLA.0000000000001694.
2. Bonadio W, Brazg J, Telt N, Pe M, Doss F, Dancy L, et al. Impact of in-hospital timing to appendectomy on perforation rates in children with appendicitis. J Emerg Med. 2015;49(5):597–604.
3. Meltzer JA, Kunkov S, Chao JH, Tay ET, George JP, Borukhov D, et al. Association of delay in appendectomy with perforation in children with appendicitis. Pediatr Emerg Care. 2016;30(10):0000000000000850.
4. Stevenson MD, Dayan PS, Dudley NC, Bajaj L, Macias CG, Bachur RG, et al. Time from emergency department evaluation to operation and appendiceal perforation. Pediatrics. 2017;139(6). https://doi.org/10.1542/peds.2016-0742. Epub 2017 May 24.
5. Gaskill CE, Simianu VV, Carnell J, Hippe DS, Bhargava P, Flum DR, et al. Use of computed tomography to determine perforation in patients with acute appendicitis. Curr Probl Diagn Radiol. 2018;47(1):6–9. https://doi.org/10.1067/j.cpradiol.2016.12.002. Epub Dec 7.
6. Kim MS, Park HW, Park JY, Park HJ, Lee SY, Hong HP, et al. Differentiation of early perforated from nonperforated appendicitis: MDCT findings, MDCT diagnostic performance, and clinical outcome. Abdom Imaging. 2014;39(3):459–66. https://doi.org/10.1007/s00261-014-0117-x.
7. Verma R, Grechushkin V, Carter D, Barish M, Pryor A, Telem D. Use and accuracy of computed tomography scan in diagnosing perforated appendicitis. Am Surg. 2015;81(4):404–7.
8. Anandalwar SP, Cameron DB, Graham DA, Melvin P, Dunlap JL, Kashtan M, et al. Association of intraoperative findings with outcomes and resource use in children with complicated appendicitis. JAMA Surg. 2018;25:2689032.
9. Boomer LA, Cooper JN, Anandalwar S, Fallon SC, Ostlie D, Leys CM, et al. Delaying appendectomy does not lead to higher rates of surgical site infections: a multi-institutional

analysis of children with appendicitis. Ann Surg. 2016;264(1):164–8. https://doi.org/10.1097/SLA.0000000000001396.

10. Serres SK, Cameron DB, Glass CC, Graham DA, Zurakowski D, Karki M, et al. Time to appendectomy and risk of complicated appendicitis and adverse outcomes in children. JAMA Pediatr. 2017;171(8):740–6. https://doi.org/10.1001/jamapediatrics.2017.0885.

11. Serres SK, Graham DA, Glass CC, Cameron DB, Anandalwar SP, Rangel SJ. Influence of time to appendectomy and operative duration on hospital cost in children with uncomplicated appendicitis. J Am Coll Surg. 2018;226(6):1014–21. https://doi.org/10.1016/j.jamcollsurg.2017.11.004. Epub Nov 16.

12. Boomer LA, Cooper JN, Deans KJ, et al. Does delay in appendectomy affect surgical site infection in children with appendicitis? J Pediatr Surg. 2014;49(6):1026–1029; discussion 1029.

13. Gurien LA, Wyrick DL, Smith SD, Dassinger MS. Optimal timing of appendectomy in the pediatric population. J Surg Res. 2016;202(1):126–31.

14. Mandeville K, Monuteaux M, Pottker T, Bulloch B. Effects of timing to diagnosis and appendectomy in pediatric appendicitis. Pediatr Emerg Care. 2015;31(11):753–8.

15. Yardeni D, Hirschl RB, Drongowski RA, Teitelbaum DH, Geiger JD, Coran AG. Delayed versus immediate surgery in acute appendicitis: do we need to operate during the night? J Pediatr Surg. 2004;39(3):464–469; discussion 464–469.

Surgical Techniques in Pediatric Appendectomy

11

Natasha R. Ahuja and David H. Rothstein

Introduction

Currently, there are four common techniques used for appendectomy: open, laparoscopic, single-incision laparoscopic surgery (SILS), and transumbilical laparoscopic-assisted appendectomy (TULAA). For the sake of completeness, we will also include natural orifice transluminal endoscopic surgery (NOTES), although this technique has not been used in pediatric patients. The operations will be described in detail along with advantages and disadvantages for each. Differences in cost, operative time, hospital recovery time, cosmetic appearance, and outcomes will be taken into account, as all of these aspects are commonly used to determine which technique is most effective in a given patient population.

Discussion

Open Technique

The first appendectomy was reported in 1735 by Claudius Amyand, who operated on an 11-year-old boy when the child perforated his appendix by swallowing a pin [1]. A century later, Charles McBurney, an American surgeon, popularized his classic

N. R. Ahuja
Department of Surgery, University at Buffalo Jacobs School of Medicine and Biomedical Sciences, Buffalo, NY, USA

D. H. Rothstein (✉)
Department of Surgery, University at Buffalo Jacobs School of Medicine and Biomedical Sciences, Buffalo, NY, USA

Department of Pediatric Surgery, John R. Oishei Children's Hospital, Buffalo, NY, USA
e-mail: drothstein@kaleidahealth.org

© Springer Nature Switzerland AG 2019
C. J. Hunter (ed.), *Controversies in Pediatric Appendicitis*,
https://doi.org/10.1007/978-3-030-15006-8_11

McBurney's incision, which allowed access to the right iliac fossa through a muscle-splitting and muscle-sparing technique to remove the appendix [1]. In this open approach, an incision is made in the right lower quadrant, superior to the inguinal ligament, parallel to the fibers of the external oblique muscle, allowing the muscle to be spared and thus speeding up the healing process. The cecum is visualized and the appendix is located, secured, and amputated at the base [2]. Other incisions may be used for an open appendectomy, such as the Rocky-Davis, a transverse incision, or a conservative midline incision, but these incisions cut through muscle and are therefore associated with increased pain and longer recuperation.

Open appendectomy may be performed quickly and is not very resource intensive, as it requires little other than retractors and basic suture material. Worldwide, the technique is practiced by a variety of surgical and nonsurgical providers. The operation can be done under general, regional, or even local anesthesia if necessary. Based on a large meta-analysis study, the average operating time for an open appendectomy is typically 11.5 minutes shorter than laparoscopic surgery, although this is surgeon-dependent [3]. Disadvantages include lack of clear visualization of peritoneal areas outside of the right iliac fossa and a visible scar. For example, in the case of misdiagnosis of appendicitis, examination of the ovaries in a female patient through the right lower quadrant incision is nearly impossible. In the United States, open appendectomy in the pediatric population has been supplanted by any one of a number of laparoscopic approaches as these offer decreased pain, less scarring, and, a potentially, faster recovery [4].

Laparoscopic Technique

The first laparoscopic appendectomy was reported in 1982, and this approach has become the gold standard for acute appendicitis management due to decreased postoperative pain, shorter hospital stay, and better cosmesis [1, 4]. One port is placed in the umbilicus, which is used to explore the peritoneal cavity and confirm the diagnosis of acute appendicitis [2, 5]. The ease of confirming the diagnosis is a major advantage of laparoscopic surgery over an open technique. Two additional ports, typically placed in the left lower quadrant and suprapubic areas, allow placement of working instruments. The mesoappendix is secured by staples or electrocautery, and a linear stapling device or endoloop is used to secure the base of the appendix. The appendix is then removed, often after placing it into a plastic bag endoscopically [2]. Endoloop closures appear to have outcomes comparable to those of a stapling device vis-à-vis operative time and safety, but are markedly cheaper [6]. Some surgeons prefer the stapler due to its ease of application and in cases where the base of the appendix is thickened or friable [2].

Innumerable studies have attempted to compare open to laparoscopic surgery in terms of operative times and costs, incidence of wound and organ space infection, pain control, and hospital stay. Meta-analyses comparing the two techniques generally suggest that laparoscopic surgery is more expensive but faster than open surgery, especially with increased practice, and results in shorter hospital lengths of stay and reduced incidences of superficial wound infections [3, 7]. Most studies also suggest that there is a slightly higher rate of intra-abdominal infections following laparoscopic surgery for perforated appendicitis in comparison to open surgery, but these associations are less uniform [8].

Large single-center observational studies and national database studies have suggested that the laparoscopic approach for both simple and perforated appendicitis is more expensive than open but otherwise has comparable or better outcomes in terms of the above measures and leads to less postoperative pain and earlier discharge [7, 9]. No randomized control study, however, has been carried out to help prove causality, and none is likely to occur as laparoscopy has become the preferred approach among pediatric surgeons in the United States. Even in the past 5 years, techniques and approaches continue to be refined in an effort to decrease cost and shorten hospital length of stay [10, 11].

Single-Incision Laparoscopic Surgery (SILS)

Recently, single-incision laparoscopic surgery (SILS) has been introduced to the pediatric population and has shown to be equal to the conventional three-trocar laparoscopic technique [4, 5]. A 2 or 3 cm port is placed into the umbilicus, and all the tools are used through this single port. This technique requires advanced laparoscopic skills as multiple tools placed through one port can lead to instrument clashing inside and outside the abdomen. Visualization and tissue manipulation are more difficult within one port, and the operation can be more time-consuming than conventional laparoscopic surgery, particularly early in the learning curve [4, 12]. Furthermore, placement of a second port is sometimes required to allow for easier dissection and triangulation. Maintaining cosmetic advantages and decreasing pain over the three-trocar approaches takes learning as well [13]. However, with practice, these disadvantages can significantly improve over time [13, 14].

With the advancement to SILS, surgeons have been concerned about the outcomes and costs that come along with this procedure compared to traditional laparoscopic procedures. In comparing the two techniques, Wieck et al. found that in non-perforated appendicitis, SILS had significant shorter operative times, decreased costs, and shorter hospital stays. Even more so, there was no difference in the rate of wound infection or abscess formation regardless of appendicitis severity [15, 16]. In addition, postoperative analgesic requirements were equivalent, but the SILS technique was felt to have a better cosmetic outcome [15, 17].

Other studies that have shown SILS take longer time in the OR by just a few minutes, which leads to greater charges. However, they still have similar postoperative morbidity and wound infection rates [16, 18]. At this time, there is no randomized, prospective study that has compared the outcomes of SILS and laparoscopic surgery.

Transumbilical Laparoscopic-Assisted Appendectomy (TULAA)

TULAA is a further advancement in the various techniques to surgically manage acute appendicitis, first successfully completed by Pelosi in 1992 [19]. This technique combines the methods of open and single-port laparoscopic surgeries as a single port is placed in the umbilicus to explore the peritoneal cavity and visualize the appendix. One can use a specialized port originally developed by gynecologists that has an offset camera lens or a conventional 12 mm port that allows placement of a grasping instrument alongside the camera lens (Fig. 11.1). The appendiceal tip is grasped and brought into the wound, allowing extracorporeal division of the mesoappendix and ligation of the appendiceal base (Fig. 11.2) [19, 20].

While the method may seem more complicated than the other techniques discussed thus far, it has been found to have many advantages. Primarily, it has been found to have shorter operative times compared to laparoscopic appendectomies, 33 minutes compared to 39 minutes in one study [20]. Operative costs for TULAA are markedly less compared to laparoscopic surgeries, in part due to the shorter operative times as well as the decreased reliance on disposable items. For example, TULAA uses an absorbable suture rather than staples or endoloops for appendiceal base control and does not require an endocatch bag; these savings can approach $1000 per case [19, 21, 22].

Even when removing the appendix extracorporeally, there has been no increase in the rate of complications and wound infections [18, 23] (Fig. 11.3). Similarly, the cosmetic results have been found to be better than the other techniques [23, 24]. Some studies have found TULAA to be a practical alternative to conventional laparoscopic or open appendectomy [24, 25].

Fig. 11.1 Instruments placed side by side in single-port transumbilical operation

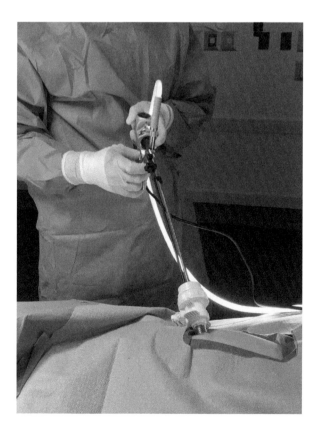

Fig. 11.2 Appendix grasped intracorporeally

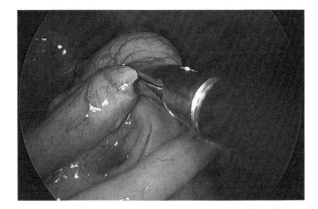

Fig. 11.3 Extracorporeal ligation of appendiceal base

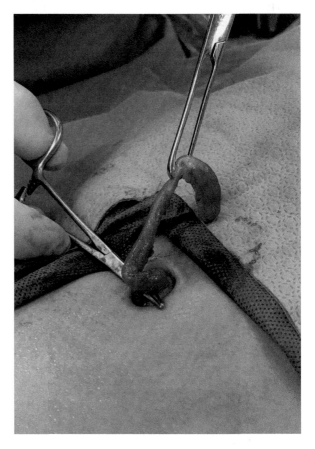

However, there are some disadvantages to TULAA. Primarily, there is a steep learning curve. Using a single port can be difficult for new users as there is increased possibility of "tool clashing" [18]. Second, while using TULAA, there are situations where it is not safe to continue with one port, in which cases a second port needed to be added, therefore, adding a second scar for the patient. Visnjic et al. found that a second port was required in 3–7% of cases, typically for complicated appendicitis [20]. With practice and time, these disadvantages can also improve.

Natural Orifice Transluminal Endoscopic Surgery (NOTES)

While SILS and TULAA are considered essentially "scarless" as there is only a transumbilical incision that is hidden within the umbilicus, surgeons continue to search for a way to remove the appendix without any skin incision. Transgastric and transvaginal appendectomies have been described in adults, although the operation often requires placement of a small umbilical assist trocar [26]. Given the ease and overall low complication rate of transumbilical surgery, as well as the slow adoption of NOTES appendectomy in adult surgery, there has been very little interest generated in pediatric NOTES appendectomy to date [27]. As instrument miniaturization evolves, NOTES techniques may someday be popularized, at least in older pediatric patients.

NOTES requires specialized tools, which may also play into part the slow adoption of this technique in both adult and pediatric populations. There is an adaption to NOTES that has been developed to make a single incision while using the endoscope, known as single-incision pediatric endoscopic surgery (SIPES) [28]. This technique still offers essentially a scarless surgery and offers a more broad application. However, there are still some disadvantages with SIPES as exposure can be challenging and instruments clash within the single site. Table 11.1 summarizes the advantages and disadvantages of the various approaches.

Table 11.1 Comparison of appendectomy techniques

Techniques	Advantages	Disadvantages
Open	Full exposure, rule out gynecological pathology, shorter operative time, conventional and more easily available tools	Typically more postoperative pain, larger scar, longer hospital stay
Laparoscopic	Decreased pain, improved cosmesis due to smaller incisions, shorter hospital stay, conventional tools, perhaps lower risk of intra-abdominal adhesions	Greater number of scars, increased costs, longer operative time
SILS	Improved cosmesis (essentially scarless) as port is through umbilicus, shorter operative time, quicker return to physical activity, conventional tools	Advanced skills needed, can hit tools unknowingly, expensive
TULAA	Safe, effective, basically scarless, combines open and laparoscopic advantages, shorter operative time, low complications rate, excellent cosmetic results	Learning curve
NOTES	Scarless, quicker return of bowel function, decreased post-op pain	Not yet developed for use in children, expensive, difficult to maneuver, sometimes needs a port in umbilicus – adding a scar

Conclusion

Laparoscopic appendectomy has generally replaced open appendectomy in the pediatric population, although the latter is still used in rural parts of the country where adult surgeons may provide a majority of pediatric surgical care. Conventional, three-port laparoscopic surgery and its subsequent single site surgery iterations appear to be quicker and associated with fewer complications when compared to open surgery, at an increased operative cost.

Clinical Pearls

- Laparoscopic appendectomy has become the preferred method for treating pediatric appendicitis as it has shorter operative time, shorter hospital stays, decreased postoperative pain, and decreased incidence of superficial wound infections.
- TULAA allows for combining open and laparoscopic techniques, which has led to no increase in wound infections and complications, shorter operative times, and decreased operative costs compared to laparoscopic surgery.
- NOTES allows for a scarless surgery but requires highly specialized tools that will need to be developed specifically for the pediatric population.

References

1. Prystowsky JB, Pugh CM, Nagle AP. Appendicitis. Curr Probl Surg. 2005;42:688–742.
2. Townsend CM, Beauchamp RD, Evers BM, Mattox KL. Sabiston textbook of surgery. 20th ed. Philadelphia: Elsevier; 2017.
3. Dai L, Shuai J. Laparoscopic versus open appendectomy in adults and children: a meta-analysis of randomized controlled trials. United European Gastroenterol J. 2017;5(4):542–53.
4. Burjonrappa SC, Nerkar H. Teaching single-incision laparoscopic appendectomy in pediatric patients. JSLS. 2012;16:619–22.
5. Raakow R, Jacob DA. Initial experience in laparoscopic single-port appendectomy: a pilot study. Dig Surg. 2011;28:74–9.
6. Parikh PP, Tashiro J, Wagenaar AE, Curbelo M, Perez EA, Neville HL. Looped suture versus stapler device in pediatric laparoscopic appendectomy: a comparative outcomes and intraoperative cost analysis. J Pediatr Surg. 2018;53:616–9.
7. Aziz O, Athanasiou T, Tekkis PP, Purkayastha S, Haddow J, Malinovski V, Paraskeva P, Darzi A. Laparoscopic versus open appendectomy in children: a meta-analysis. Ann Surg. 2006;243(1):17–27.
8. Zhang S, Du T, Jiang X, Song C. Laparoscopic appendectomy in children with perforated appendicitis: a meta-analysis. Surg Laparosc Endosc Percutan Tech. 2017;27(4):262–6.
9. Jen HC, Shew SB. Laparoscopic versus open appendectomy in children: outcomes comparison based on statewide analysis. J Surg Res. 2010;161:13–7.
10. Grewal H, Sweat J, Vazquez WD. Laparoscopic appendectomy in children can be done as a fast-track or same-day surgery. JSLS. 2004;8(2):151–4.
11. Cairo SB, Raval MV, Browne MB, Meyers H, Rothstein DH. Association of same-day discharge with hospital readmission after appendectomy in pediatric patients. JAMA Surg. 2017. https://doi.org/10.1001/jamasurg.2017.2221.

12. Rothenberg SS, Shipman K, Yoder S. Experience with modified single-port laparoscopic procedures in children. J Laparoendosc Adv Surg Tech. 2009;19:695–9.
13. Oltmann SC, Garcia NM, Ventura B, Mitchell I, Fischer AC. Single-incision laparoscopic surgery: feasibility for pediatric appendectomies. J Pediatr Surg. 2010;45:1208–12.
14. Dutta S. Early experience with single incision laparoscopic surgery: eliminating the scar from abdominal operations. J Pediatr Surg. 2009;44:1741–5.
15. Wieck MM, Hamilton NA, Krishnaswami S. A cost and outcome analysis of pediatric single-incision appendectomy. J Surg Res. 2016;203:253–7.
16. Antoniou SA, Koch OO, Antoniou GA, Lasithiotakis K, Chalkiadakis GE, Pointner R, Granderath FA. Meta-analysis of randomized trials on single-incision laparoscopic versus conventional laparoscopic appendectomy. Am J Surg. 2014;207:613–22.
17. Ahmed K, Wang TT, Patel VM, Nagpal K, Clark J, Ali M, et al. The role of single-incision laparoscopic surgery in abdominal and pelvic surgery: a systemic review. Surg Endosc. 2011;25:378–96.
18. Frutos MD, Abrisqueta J, Lujan J, Abellan I, Parrilla P. Randomized prospective study to compare laparoscopic appendectomy versus umbilical single-incision appendectomy. Ann Surg. 2013;257:413–8.
19. Perin G, Scarpa MG. TULAA: a minimally invasive appendectomy technique for the pediatric patient. Minim Invasive Surg. 2016. https://doi.org/10.1155/2016/6132741.
20. Visnjic S. Transumbilical laparoscopically assisted appendectomy in children: high-tech low-budget surgery. Surg Endosc. 2008;22:1667–71.
21. Munakata K, Uemura M, Shimizu J, Miyake M, Hata T, Ikeda K, et al. Gasless transumbilical laparoscopic-assisted appendectomy as a safe and cost-effective alternative surgical procedure for mild acute appendicitis. Surg Today. 2016;46:319–25.
22. Kulaylat AN, Podany AB, Holenbeak CS, Santaos MC, Rocourt DV. Transumbilical laparoscopic-assisted appendectomy is associated with lower costs compared to multiport laparoscopic appendectomy. J Pediatr Surg. 2014;49:1508–12.
23. Noviello C, Romano M, Martino A, Cobellis G. Transumbilical laparoscopic-assisted appendectomy in the treatment of acute uncomplicated appendicitis in children. Gastroenterol Res Pract. 2015. https://doi.org/10.1155/2015/949162.
24. Pappalepore N, Tursini S, Marino N, Lisi G, Lelli Chiesa P. Transumbilical laparoscopic-assisted appendectomy (TULAA): a safe and useful alternative for uncomplicated appendicitis. Eur J Pediatr Surg. 2002;12:383–6.
25. Stanfill AB, Matilsky DK, Kalvakuri K, Pearl RH, Wallace LJ, Vegunta RK. Transumbilical laparoscopically assisted appendectomy: an alternative minimally invasive technique in pediatric patients. J Laparoendosc Adv Surg Tech. 2010;20:873–6.
26. Isaza N, Garcia P, Dutta S. Advances in pediatric minimal access therapy: a cautious journey from therapeutic endoscopy to transluminal surgery based on the adult experience. J Pediatr Gastroenterol Nutr. 2008;46:359–69.
27. Thomson M. Natural orifice transluminal endoscopic surgery for the antireflux process in children. Tech Gastrointest Endosc. 2013;15:52–5.
28. Hansen EN, Muensterer OJ, Georgeson KE, Harmon CM. Single-incision pediatric endosurgery: lessons learned from our first 224 laparoendoscopic single-site procedures in children. Pediatr Surg Int. 2011;27:643–8.

The Controversial Role of Interval Appendectomy

12

Alexander W. Peters and Demetri J. Merianos

Case Example

An 11-year-old male with no past medical history presents to the local emergency room with 5 days of worsening abdominal pain, nausea, vomiting, and fevers. On abdominal exam, he has a tender mass in the right lower quadrant. He has a leukocytosis of 15,000, and on ultrasound he has a right lower quadrant phlegmon from presumed complicated appendicitis. He is admitted to the pediatric ward for intravenous antibiotics, and his symptoms resolve within a few days. He is discharged after 5 days and completes an additional 10 days of oral antibiotic therapy. At his 1 month follow-up appointment, he reports no further issues and has returned to all of his normal activities, including sports. His parents ask you if he needs to have his appendix removed. What would you recommend?

Introduction

Interval appendectomy is defined as removal of the appendix after successful non-operative management of acute appendicitis. Traditionally, interval appendectomy refers specifically to removal of the appendix after resolution of complicated, or perforated, appendicitis, typically associated with an appendiceal mass or abscess. However, with the increase in non-operative management of uncomplicated appendicitis, surgeons may be faced with this decision after non-operative management of uncomplicated appendicitis as well.

A. W. Peters · D. J. Merianos (✉)
Department of Surgery, Division of Pediatric Surgery, New York-Presbyterian/ Weill Cornell Medical Center, New York, NY, USA
e-mail: dem9110@med.cornell.edu

© Springer Nature Switzerland AG 2019
C. J. Hunter (ed.), *Controversies in Pediatric Appendicitis*,
https://doi.org/10.1007/978-3-030-15006-8_12

Discussion

Uncomplicated Appendicitis

Since the stated rationale for non-operative management of uncomplicated appendicitis is to avoid surgery altogether, one can presume that most surgeons favoring interval appendectomy for uncomplicated appendicitis would have instead chosen early appendectomy at initial presentation. However, parents who initially agreed to non-operative management of uncomplicated appendicitis may later seek definitive treatment, especially if their child has further bouts of abdominal pain after discharge.

The decision regarding whether or not to perform an interval appendectomy is largely based on the evidence-based observation, or more often the perception, of the risk of recurrent appendicitis compared to the risks associated with interval appendectomy. Several studies have looked at the rate of recurrent appendicitis after non-operative management of uncomplicated appendicitis, with recurrence rates ranging from 24% to 38% [1–3].

Perioperative complication rates for interval appendectomy after successful non-operative management of uncomplicated appendicitis can be presumed to be as low, or lower than, complication rates after early appendectomy for uncomplicated appendicitis, because the surgeon is less likely to encounter active inflammation during the interval procedure. Therefore, the argument against interval appendectomy following successful non-operative management of uncomplicated appendicitis is similar to the initial argument in favor of non-operative management of uncomplicated appendicitis. Surgeons must weigh the global risk reduction and cost savings of removing 24–38 appendices per 100 patients with acute recurrent appendicitis, against removing all 100 appendices up front, or in a controlled, elective, interval setting.

Complicated Appendicitis

The rate of complicated appendicitis in children is estimated to range from 10% to 30% [4], with the term "complicated appendicitis" encompassing ruptured or perforated appendices, in addition to appendiceal abscess, phlegmon, or inflammatory mass. The vast majority of interval appendectomies are performed 2–3 months after an episode of complicated appendicitis, in patients whose initial episode has been successfully managed non-operatively. The rationale for non-operative initial management of these patients is the fear of higher complication rates (risk of enterotomy, need for ileocecectomy, etc.) during early appendectomy in the setting of intense intra-abdominal inflammation. While there is significant debate regarding the optimal management of these patients, with some surgeons advocating for early appendectomy, for the purposes of this chapter, we will consider only patients who are successfully managed non-operatively and who are then candidates for elective, interval appendectomy.

Table 12.1 Rate of recurrent appendicitis after non-operative management of complicated appendicitis

	Non-operative management	Recurrent appendicitis
Puapong et al. [5]	$N = 61$, 7.5 year F/U	$N = 5$ (8%)
Svensson et al. [6]	$N = 89$, 5.1 year F/U	$N = 9$ (10%)
Ein et al. [7]	$N = 49$, 7 year F/U	$N = 21$ (43%)
Fawkner-Corbett et al. [8]	$N = 69$, 3 month F/U	$N = 8$ (12%)
Tanaka et al. [9]	$N = 38$, 3.3 year F/U	$N = 13$ (34.2%)

As with uncomplicated appendicitis, our decision regarding whether or not to perform interval appendectomy again begins with an analysis of the risk of recurrent appendicitis versus the risks associated with interval appendectomy. Historically, all patients who were managed non-operatively for complicated appendicitis were recommended to have interval appendectomy, as the risk of recurrent appendicitis was presumed to be high; however, this practice has been called into question over the past decade. Several studies have sought to determine the rate of recurrent appendicitis after non-operative management of complicated appendicitis, with recurrence rates ranging from 8% to 43% [5–9] (see Table 12.1).

In 2007, Puapong et al. followed 72 patients with complicated appendicitis managed non-operatively, for a mean of 7.5 years, 61 of whom did not undergo interval appendectomy. Of those 61 patients, 5 (8%) developed recurrent appendicitis, with 80% of those recurrences occurring within 6 months of the initial episode [5].

A more recent study by Svensson et al. followed 89 patients for a mean of 5.1 years, after successful non-operative management of complicated appendicitis. A total of 12 patients (13%) were readmitted, and 9 patients (10%) underwent unplanned interval appendectomy, 2 for recurrent appendicitis, 2 for readmission with an abscess, 3 for readmission without an abscess, and 2 for parental request. In addition, there were 29 patients (33%) seen in the emergency department who did not require surgical intervention, but they did have a total of 21 imaging studies [6].

Ein et al. followed 96 pediatric patients with complicated appendicitis for a mean of 7 years, with 49 patients being successfully managed non-operatively, without planned interval appendectomy. Of these, 21 patients (43%) developed recurrent appendicitis, often within 3 months of the initial episode [7].

Lacking large-scale, prospective trials, a systematic review of three studies ($n = 127$) performed by Hall et al. calculated an overall 20.5% incidence of recurrent appendicitis after successful non-operative management of complicated appendicitis [10]. Interestingly, these rates are similar to rates of recurrent appendicitis after uncomplicated appendicitis, which is supported by histopathologic analysis of interval appendectomy specimens after complicated appendicitis, showing that previously perforated appendices do not generally have an obliterated lumen [11]. Thus, there is no reason to think that the risk of recurrent appendicitis would be different after complicated appendicitis, as compared to uncomplicated appendicitis.

However, it is widely believed that complication rates after interval appendectomy for complicated appendicitis are significantly higher than complication rates after interval appendectomy for uncomplicated appendicitis, due to the existence of intra-abdominal adhesions, scarring, and occasionally smoldering inflammation, after complicated appendicitis. While historical complication rates are reported to be as high as 23% [12], the previously mentioned systematic review by Hall et al. analyzed 23 studies ($n = 1247$) for complication rates associated with interval appendectomy after successful non-operative treatment of appendiceal mass and found the overall incidence to be only 3.4% [10].

Appendicolith

Several studies have identified the presence of an appendicolith as an independent risk factor for failure of non-operative management of children with both uncomplicated and complicated appendicitis. In the previously mentioned study by Ein et al., the presence of an appendicolith was associated with a 72% rate of recurrent appendicitis, compared with a 26% recurrence rate in those patients who did not have an appendicolith [7]. In a study by Tanaka et al., 47% (9/19) of patients with an appendicolith failed non-operative management, compared to 24% (14/59) of patients without an appendicolith ($p = 0.05$) [2].

An additional study by Zhang et al. showed that the risk of recurrent appendicitis after non-operative management of complicated appendicitis was approximately twice as high (19%) in children with appendicolith, as compared to children without appendicolith (9%) [13]. Finally, a recent prospective trial in the United States that evaluated non-operative management of uncomplicated appendicitis in children with an appendicolith was terminated early due to high failure rate of non-operative management [14]. Therefore, most authors recommend that patients with an appendicolith in the setting of complicated appendicitis should be offered interval appendectomy and most protocols for non-operative management of uncomplicated appendicitis exclude patients with appendicoliths.

Histopathology

Another variable affecting the decision to perform interval appendectomy is the ability to diagnose neuroendocrine (carcinoid) tumors, or other significant pathologies, such as granulomatous appendicitis as the initial presentation of Crohn's disease. Non-operative management without interval appendectomy precludes histopathological inspection of the appendix, which has been shown to contain a neuroendocrine tumor in 0.3–0.8% of pediatric patients [15]. Similarly, the previously mentioned systematic review by Hall et al. examined 15 studies ($n = 955$) and reports the incidence of carcinoid tumors to be 0.9% [10]. Other diagnoses, such as right ovarian torsion, or Meckel's diverticulitis, are also occasionally diagnosed during surgical exploration for suspected appendicitis, but these entities are considered less likely to be missed with advances in radiology and other modern diagnostics.

Conclusion

In summary, despite several studies evaluating the role of interval appendectomy, the procedure remains controversial. Although complications associated with elective interval appendectomy are minimal, complications associated with emergent appendectomy for recurrent appendicitis also remain low, and at least two studies suggest that recurrences may present with more mild clinical symptoms [9, 16]. Therefore, given the relatively low risk of recurrent appendicitis, several studies have come to the conclusion that interval appendectomy may not be necessary.

Nevertheless, while there seems to be consensus in favor of interval appendectomy in the setting of a known appendicolith, conclusive data for most other questions remains elusive. While the data broadly suggests that interval appendectomy may represent an avoidable expense from a health system perspective, interval appendectomy may still save many patients the inconvenience of unplanned ER visits, readmissions, emergency surgery, and, in rare cases, missed or delayed diagnoses of other significant pathologies. Therefore, pediatric surgeons must carefully weigh any decision to pursue or refrain from interval appendectomy following successful non-operative therapy within the context of each individual patient. Figure 12.1 illustrates a proposed treatment algorithm, based on currently available data.

Regardless of our personal beliefs or preferences, as pediatric surgeons, we have an ethical and moral obligation to disclose the risks, benefits, and probabilities to our patients and their families and ensure that whatever decision is made regarding the management of their child is made in the best interests of the child. However, as healthcare providers we are also stewards of healthcare expenditures, and we have an additional ethical and moral obligation to reduce spending in instances where no proven benefit exists to support a more expensive therapy.

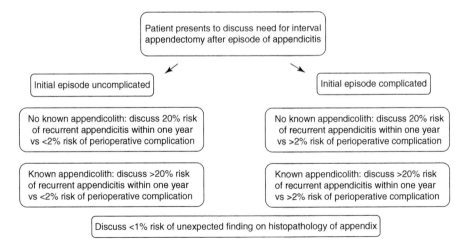

Fig. 12.1 Proposed treatment algorithm for discussing the merits of interval appendectomy with patients and their parents

Therefore, it appears that the challenge in deciding whether or not to recommend interval appendectomy lies not in the data itself but rather in the lens through which it is viewed. Is a 20% rate of recurrent appendicitis considered a failure in 20% of patients who otherwise could have had their disease surgically cured at their initial presentation, or does it represent a triumph in the 80% of children who were spared an unnecessary operation? This ideological struggle is well illustrated by the title of a recent study by Tanaka et al. [9], which asks the following question: "More than one-third of successfully non-operatively treated patients with complicated appendicitis experienced recurrent appendicitis: Is interval appendectomy necessary?" It depends on how we define "successfully treated." Either way, the decision to pursue interval appendectomy in pediatric patients is complex and, in lieu of clearer data, must be carefully weighed in the context of every child.

Clinical Pearls

- Interval appendectomy may be preferable in cases where a fecolith is identified.
- A balanced discussion of the pros and cons of interval appendectomy is needed on a case-by-case basis.

References

1. Svensson JF, Patkova B, Almstrom M, et al. Nonoperative treatment with antibiotics versus surgery for acute nonperforated appendicitis in children: a pilot randomized controlled trial. Ann Surg. 2015;261(1):67–71.
2. Tanaka Y, Uchida H, Kawashima H, et al. Long-term outcomes of operative versus nonoperative treatment for uncomplicated appendicitis. J Pediatr Surg. 2015;50(11):1893–7.
3. Minneci PC, Lodwick DL, Sulkowski JP, et al. The effectiveness of patient choice in nonoperative versus surgical management of uncomplicated acute appendicitis. JAMA Surg. 2016;151(5):408–15.
4. Andersson RE, Petzold MG. Nonsurgical treatment of appendiceal abscess or phlegmon: a systematic review and meta-analysis. Ann Surg. 2007;246:741–8.
5. Puapong D, Lee SL, Haigh PI, Kaminski A, Liu I-LA, Applebaum H. Routine interval appendectomy in children is not indicated. J Pediatr Surg. 2007;42(9):1500–3.
6. Svensson JF, Johansson R, Kaiser S, Wester T. Recurrence of acute appendicitis after nonoperative treatment of appendiceal abscess in children: a single-centre experience. Pediatr Surg Int. 2014;30(4):413–6.
7. Ein SH, Langer JC, Daneman A. Nonoperative management of pediatric ruptured appendix with inflammatory mass or abscess: presence of an appendicolith predicts recurrent appendicitis. J Pediatr Surg. 2005;40(10):1612–5.
8. Fawkner-Corbett D, Jawaid WB, McPartland J, Losty PD. Interval appendectomy in children clinical outcomes, financial costs and patient benefits. Pediatr Surg Int. 2014;30(7):743–6.
9. Tanaka Y, Uchida H, Kawashima H, et al. More than one-third of successfully nonoperatively treated patients with complicated appendicitis experienced recurrent appendicitis: is interval appendectomy necessary? J Pediatr Surg. 2016;51(12):1957–61.
10. Hall NJ, Jones CE, Eaton S, Stanton MP, Burge DM. Is interval appendicectomy justified after successful nonoperative treatment of an appendix mass in children? A systematic review. J Pediatr Surg. 2011;46(4):767–71.

11. Mazziotti MV, Marley EF, Winthrop AL, Fitzgerald PG, Walton M, Langer JC. Histopathologic analysis of interval appendectomy specimens: support for the role of interval appendectomy. J Pediatr Surg. 1997;32(6):806–9.
12. Lewin J, Fenyo G, Engstrom L. Treatment of appendiceal abscess. Acta Chir Scand. 1988;154:123–5.
13. Zhang HL, Bai YZ, Zhou X, Wang WL. Nonoperative treatment of appendiceal phlegmon or abscess with an appendicolith in children. J Gastrointest Surg. 2013;4:766–70.
14. Mahida JB, Lodwick DL, Nacion KM, et al. High failure rate of non-operative management of acute appendicitis with an appendicolith in children. J Pediatr Surg. 2016;51(6):908.
15. Henderson L, Fahily C, Folaranmi S, et al. Management and outcome of neuroendocrine tumours of the appendix – a two centre UK experience. J Pediatr Surg. 2014;49(10):1513–7.
16. Sakorafas GH, Sabanis D, Lappas C, et al. Interval routine appendectomy following conservative treatment of acute appendicitis: is it really needed. World J Gastrointest Surg. 2012;4(4):83–6.

Diagnostic and Management Strategies for Postoperative Complications in Pediatric Appendicitis

13

Cynthia Susai, Julie Monteagudo, and Francois I. Luks

Case Example

Six days after a laparoscopic appendectomy for perforated appendicitis and peritonitis, a 12-year-old male is finally tolerating sips of clear liquids. His maximal temperature has decreased from 103 °F (39.4 °C) on postoperative day 2 to 101.5 °F (38.6 °C). He still has abdominal tenderness, although he is less distended than before, and he is passing flatus. He had one episode of very loose stools.

When should he be worked up for an intra-abdominal abscess? Which factors (vital signs, laboratory tests, and other findings) would be the most reliable indicators of an infectious complications, if any? When and how would you image him?

Introduction

The overall complication rate from appendicitis ranges between 10% and 15% [1, 2]. Most complications are infectious in nature, ranging from superficial wound infections to intra-abdominal and pelvic abscesses. The exact risk depends on the disease process: while early uncomplicated appendicitis has complication rates ranging from 1% to 7%, these rates increase up to 30% in the presence of perforation and peritonitis [3, 4]. Similarly, non-perforated gangrenous appendicitis poses a greater risk of postoperative surgical site infection and intra-abdominal abscesses than simple appendicitis [5]. Other factors associated with the development of postoperative complications include the urgent nature of the intervention, the inherent risk of anesthesia, and the risks of the intervention itself.

C. Susai · J. Monteagudo · F. I. Luks (✉)
Division of Pediatric Surgery, Warren Alpert Medical School of Brown University, Hasbro Children's Hospital, Providence, RI, USA
e-mail: Francois_Luks@brown.edu

© Springer Nature Switzerland AG 2019
C. J. Hunter (ed.), *Controversies in Pediatric Appendicitis*,
https://doi.org/10.1007/978-3-030-15006-8_13

Predicting Postoperative Complications

Preoperative Risk Factors

The most important predictor of postoperative complications is preoperative status of the appendix, i.e., the presence or absence of perforation. However, other preoperative factors can influence the outcome, either independently or by increasing the risk of perforation. Frequently cited risk factors include age and body mass index. Appendicitis is much less common in very young children (under 5 years) than in school-age children, but when it occurs it is most often in an advanced state [6]. Reasons include a less reliable history of periumbilical pain, migrating to the right lower quadrant [7, 8]; scant omentum, which in older children and adults tends to home in on the inflammatory process, protecting the remainder of the peritoneal cavity [9]; and its rarity, leading care providers to think of other conditions first [10]. Overweight children may have an increased risk of presenting in advanced stages of appendicitis [11] and have a higher inherent risk of postoperative complications, including wound infections and respiratory problems [12, 13]. However, underweight children are also at risk, with higher rates of misdiagnosis, longer hospital length of stay, and more postoperative complications compared with children of normal weight [14].

Many researchers have examined whether race and ethnicity [15–18], socioeconomic status [15, 16], geography [19], insurance status [20], or other epidemiologic factors affect access to care and, by extension, complication rate as it relates to advanced disease. Results are conflicting, but delay of care for any reasons correlates with an increased rate of complications [21].

Other indicators are not independent risk factors but purportedly predict the presence of advanced disease and perforation. These include preoperative leukocytosis, preoperative diarrhea, delay in presentation, and risk of perforation [22–25]. Overall, factors that suggest advanced disease are of academic interest only, since most children undergo preoperative imaging, which better demonstrates the severity of appendicitis.

Intraoperative Risk Factors

Appendectomy, as any surgery, involves risks inherent to the operation itself. If it is performed as an emergency, appendectomy places the patient at risk for aspiration pneumonitis on induction of anesthesia in the presence of a full stomach. Of note, delaying surgery, as long as it occurs within 24 hours of presentation, is not associated with increased risk of complicated appendicitis or adverse outcomes [26], suggesting that appendectomy can be safely performed as an urgent procedure, rather than as an emergency. This area of controversy is discussed in more detail elsewhere in this publication. Risks associated with any operation, urgent or not, include loss of airway, cardiac arrhythmias, and, very rarely, malignant hyperthermia. Any comorbidity may of course increase these risks [27].

Variations in operative technique do not appear to affect the outcome or the risk of postoperative complications, as long as sound surgical principles are observed. Inversion of the appendiceal stump has long ago been shown to offer no advantage over simple ligation [28]; laparoscopically, stapling and ligating the appendix are equally acceptable [29, 30]. It had been suggested that the incidence of peritoneal abscesses was higher after laparoscopic than after open appendectomy for perforated appendicitis [31], but this is no longer a topic of debate [32–35]. Today, more than 85% of all appendectomies in children are performed laparoscopically [36].

Controversy surrounding peritoneal irrigation, in both simple appendicitis and diffuse peritonitis, has largely subsided. In early, suppurative appendicitis, small amounts of serous or seropurulent fluid can safely be suctioned, without the need of irrigation [37–39]. If frank purulence is present, irrigation with warmed physiologic fluid should be performed until clear return. In general, placing the patient in a reverse Trendelenburg or Fowler position promotes dependent drainage of any residual fluid toward the pelvis, facilitating postoperative drainage if an abscess were to develop [40].

Postoperative Risk Factors

Persistent fever beyond a week postoperatively, persistent or worsening nausea, vomiting, diarrhea, and abdominal pain are all signs of an infectious or obstructive complication and warrant further work-up. Any of these signs and symptoms can occur during the patient's hospitalization or after hospital discharge. Traditionally, halting antibiotic therapy or discharging a patient who has a persistent fever or leukocytosis significantly increases the risk of readmission for an infectious complication [41].

In non-perforated appendicitis, one perioperative dose of broad-spectrum antibiotics is typically enough to prevent complications such as wound infection, unless significant delay exists prior to surgery [42, 43]. For the management of perforated appendicitis, duration of postoperative intravenous antibiotic therapy should be based on clinical criteria such as abdominal pain and fever. This can be achieved with broad-spectrum single-, double-, or triple-agent therapy (although single or double agent is usually more cost-effective). Whether double pseudomonas coverage or coverage for gram-positive anaerobes such as enterococcus is necessary remains controversial [44–48]. With perforated appendicitis, intravenous antibiotics administered for less than 5 days are often supplemented with oral antibiotics for a course of 7 days [49, 50]. Finally, growing concerns about bacterial resistance to antibiotics may need to be addressed.

While it is relatively easy to identify patients who present with a complication, the difficulty lies in the *early* postoperative prediction of which patients are at a high risk of complications [51, 52]. There have been countless efforts to identify early postoperative indicators of infectious complications. To date, no reliable markers have been found. Fever on postoperative day 3 [41], leukocytosis on postoperative day 5 [25], prolonged anorexia [53], elevated serum C-reactive protein [24, 54], and appendiceal size have been cited as predictors of postoperative complications [25, 53, 55, 56]. However, most of these markers correlate with the (preoperative) extent of the disease and are therefore not independent predictors of a complication [55]. Only early postoperative diet tolerance seems to suggest an increased risk of abdominal abscess. In a recent small study of children with perforated appendicitis, none of the patients who were later found to have an abscess were tolerating a regular diet by postoperative day 3, while none of those on a regular diet developed this complication [53].

Diagnosing Postoperative Complications

Infectious Complications

Superficial SSI

These are often detected on physical exam, with pain and purulence noted along the area of the incision(s). While clinical examination is usually straightforward, ultrasonography can sometimes help identify an abdominal wall infection (deep SSI). Computed tomography (CT) can be used as well, particularly in suspected cases of deeper (intra-abdominal), as well as abdominal wall involvement. Axial imaging (ultrasound (U/S)) or CT can also help determine the integrity of the fascial closure, if it is complicated by infection [57]. The incidence of superficial SSI after perforated appendicitis was once believed to be lower after laparoscopic appendectomy than after open surgery, with rates of 1–3% [1], but there is currently no evidence that these differences, if present, are statistically significant [31].

Deep Space Infections

Deep SSI, such as an intra-abdominal abscess, should be suspected if the postoperative course is marked by persistent fevers (there is a positive correlation between abscess development and maximum daily temperature after postoperative day 3 [41]), nausea, vomiting, persistent diarrhea, dysuria or urinary retention, worsening abdominal or suprapubic pain and tenderness, and anorexia. Suspicion should be high if a patient is not tolerating a normal diet by postoperative day 5–7, and failure to resume a regular diet by postoperative day 3 may raise the suspicion of deep space infection [53]. Certainly, patients who recovered well initially and later present with any of these symptoms (during the same hospitalization or after discharge) should be worked up for a deep space infection. A higher degree of suspicion should also be prompted by risk factors such as obesity, preoperative leukocytosis >20,000/mm^3, and operative time longer than 90 minutes [12, 25, 58–60].

The timing of abscess development varies greatly between patients, but there is a continuum from postoperative fluid collections (from inflammation, residual irrigation fluid, and resuscitative efforts) to well-formed abscess, defined as a dense fluid collection surrounded by an enhancing rim (Fig. 13.1) [61]. Imaging can be obtained between postoperative days 5 and 7 to evaluate for abscess. Refraining

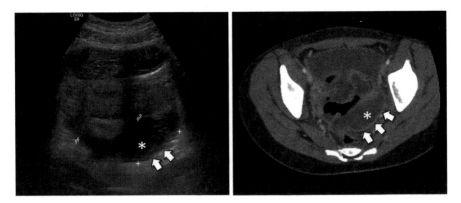

Fig. 13.1 U/S (left) and CT scan (right) images of a pelvic abscess (*). Note the hyperechoic abscess wall (arrows)

from earlier imaging (when a clear abscess wall is not yet present and spontaneous resolution can still occur) might result in fewer interventions (including CT scans and drainage procedures) without increasing adverse outcomes [62].

Other Postoperative Complications

Intestinal obstruction can be both a presenting sign of appendicitis and a postoperative complication. Peritoneal adhesions are the cause of 65–75% of all small bowel obstructions. In adults, the laparoscopic approach may reduce adhesion formation, but this finding has been challenged and has not been demonstrated in children [63]. Although the lifelong incidence of surgical intervention for adhesion-related disease is 0.8% for appendectomy [64], it is more likely to resolve with conservative measures if it occurs within the first few postoperative weeks [65]. While this complication can occur after any intra-abdominal operation, regardless of the underlying condition, intra-abdominal infections such as perforated appendicitis increase the risk of adhesive disease, certainly in the acute period. Intra-abdominal sepsis in girls is of particular concern, as it was reportedly associated with decreased fertility from pelvic scarring and adhesions [66]. That finding has been refuted in recent years, however [67].

True small bowel obstruction must be differentiated from prolonged ileus, which is not uncommon after complicated appendicitis. In the postoperative period, nausea and vomiting, especially bilious vomiting, require further investigation. A secondary ileus is often associated with too rapid diet progression. Absent bowel sounds are an indication of intestinal paralysis, and conservative treatment is warranted. Placement of a nasogastric tube is not mandatory but recommended for protracted vomiting and to ease the patient's discomfort and abdominal pain. A plain upright (or lateral decubitus) radiograph should differentiate between ileus and obstruction: the presence of differential air-fluid loops suggests an obstructive process, whereas diffusely dilated loops of small and large bowel make an ileus more likely. In case of doubt, an abdominal CT (preferably with enteric contrast) will help determine the presence of an obstruction, by demonstrating collapsed distal bowel loops, and possibly a transition point.

Clostridium difficile is an important cause of antibiotic-associated diarrhea and other manifestations of overgrowth colitis and one of the most common healthcare-associated pathogens. The manifestation of *C. difficile* can vary from asymptomatic colonization of the colon to mild diarrhea to ileus, toxic megacolon, hypotension, or shock [68]. The most common presentation of *C. difficile* is acute-onset watery diarrhea (more than three loose bowel movements a day) during or after a course of antibiotics. Severe disease may be associated with leukocytosis greater than 15,000 white blood cells/mm^3, elevated serum creatinine, hypoalbuminemia, or lactic acidosis. Laboratory testing includes polymerase chain reaction (PCR) assay for *C. difficile* toxin in a stool specimen that is loose or semi-formed [69].

Treating Postoperative Complications

Superficial SSIs

In superficial SSI, the wound must be opened and, if deep enough, irrigated and packed. In the presence of an abscess, wound drainage is sufficient therapy. If cellulitis or deeper tissue infection is present as well, broad-spectrum antibiotics may be required. In those cases, a wound culture can help guide therapy.

Historically, a contaminated or dirty wound would be left open to heal by secondary intention. The fear was that skin closure in a contaminated setting increased the risk for deeper infections, including potentially fatal necrotizing fasciitis. However, in the case of perforated appendicitis, there is no difference in superficial surgical site infections between patients who have their wound primarily closed after operation versus those that have delayed primary closure at postoperative day 3–5 [70]. It has long been established that overall patient quality of life is improved with primary closure of infected wounds, given the current incidence of wound infections requiring intervention [71].

Deep Space Infection

The management of abdominal and pelvic abscesses has dramatically changed in recent decades. While reoperation was often necessary, less invasive techniques are now commonplace and should be considered first.

Percutaneous Drain Placement

While this section addresses postoperative complications, percutaneous drainage of an appendiceal abscess can also be considered up front in selected patients with perforated appendicitis, when symptoms are relatively mild and up-front operative appendectomy might substantially worsen the patient's condition [72]. Patients with a well-circumscribed peri-appendiceal abscess can be treated with percutaneous drainage, with appendectomy generally deferred [73]. The same approach is used for postoperative abscesses. Generally, percutaneous drainage is performed in intra-abdominal abscesses greater than 2 cm in diameter. Relative contraindications for percutaneous drainage include poorly localized, loculated, complex, or diffuse fluid collections and suspicion of necrotic tissue or high density fluid, making successful drainage less likely. In these cases, or in the presence of inaccessible collections, surgical intervention may be needed. Collections smaller than 2 cm in diameter may not need to be drained and can instead be treated with antibiotics [74, 75].

According to some, percutaneous drainage under CT guidance (Fig. 13.2) has higher rates of resolution of clinical symptoms and decreased rates of recurrence than with ultrasound [76]. Thus, while ultrasound avoids radiation exposure and may be more readily available, it could have higher rates of failure and recurrence [77]. Percutaneous drainage can be performed under sedation or general anesthesia, depending on the patient's age and degree of anxiety, and on local and cultural factors at each institution. The trans-gluteal approach (Fig. 13.3) has been shown to be superior to the transabdominal approach in terms of complete resolution of clinical symptoms and decreased recurrence rates. It may also be the way to avoid injury to adjacent bowel in some cases. However, it is typically more uncomfortable or painful than other routes [76].

Although aspiration can be successful in smaller abscesses with non-thick fluid, there is moderate evidence to suggest that leaving the drain in place is more successful [78, 79]. In the presence of thick purulent drainage, daily flushing of the drainage catheter can be performed with 5–10 mL of saline, making sure to track the irrigation volume. The drain is generally left in place until drain output is minimal. Reimaging is a subject of debate and is not generally used to determine drain removal.

Transrectal Drainage

Deep pelvic abscesses that are inaccessible to percutaneous drainage may be drained transrectally. This technique has been well described since Fowler [80, 81], who

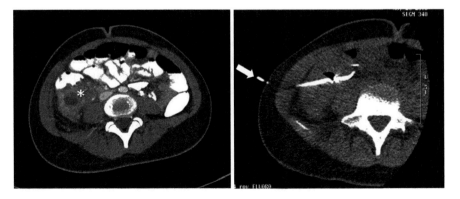

Fig. 13.2 Drainage of an intra-abdominal abscess (asterisk, left) under CT scan guidance (arrow: drain entering the right flank at the level of the umbilicus, right)

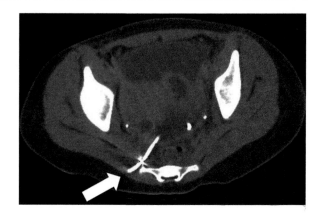

Fig. 13.3 CT scan of a trans-gluteal catheter (arrow) draining the abscess depicted in Fig. 13.1

advocated positioning a patient with peritonitis in a semi-sitting position, to effect drainage of peritoneal collections into the perirectal space – where it could more easily be accessed. With the advent of image-guided intervention, transrectal drainage has become much less common but may be the only method to access the deep pelvic collections [82], short of reoperation. For this approach, general anesthesia is typically required [83]. A retrorectal approach is the safest, to avoid other pelvic structures and vessels. The mass effect and fluctuation of the bulging abscess is determined digitally, and an incision is made at the level of the dentate line (or at the point of greatest fluctuation), draining the collection into the rectum. A soft drain can be left in place for a few days.

Operative Intervention

For very large intra-abdominal abscesses (10 cm in diameter or greater), or for complex or multiple collections not amenable to percutaneous drainage, surgical reintervention may be inevitable. Laparoscopic drainage is a minimally invasive and useful alternative to open exploration, but there is a certain risk of bowel injury secondary to postoperative adhesive changes, particularly after extensive peritonitis. It offers the advantage of exploring the abdomen and aspirating the purulent exudate under direct vision [84, 85]. However, it may be difficult to distinguish a walled-off collection from an adherent loop of intestine, and one should have a low threshold to convert to laparotomy. Copious peritoneal washout is performed after draining the abscess(es); unless there is a well-defined abscess cavity, a drain is usually not left in place.

Other Complications

C. difficile is generally treated by discontinuing the inciting antibiotic and supportive care. Either oral vancomycin or metronidazole is suggested for treatment of a first episode of non-severe *C. difficile* infection. In the case of inability to tolerate

PO, IV metronidazole or rectal vancomycin may be administered. For toxic megacolon, colonic perforation, acute abdomen, or septic shock, surgery in the form of a subtotal colectomy and diversion ileostomy may be required for lifesaving treatment [86].

The treatment of prolonged (or secondary) ileus is intestinal decompression, intravenous hydration, and patience. Early postoperative intestinal obstruction can often be treated non-operatively. However, failure to recover at all after appendectomy for perforated appendicitis should raise the suspicion of a persistent obstruction (often on a kinked intestinal loop that is involved in the inflammatory process). In that case, early diagnosis (CT scan) and surgical intervention may be warranted.

Conclusion

Although the majority of patients who undergo treatment for appendicitis fair well postoperatively, a sizeable number of individuals will experience a complicated course. The timely and accurate diagnosis of these complications and subsequent management are important in optimizing their course and improving long-term outcomes. In the case example, this patient presented several findings that concerning for complication. Firstly, he presented with a perforated appendicitis and now 6 days later continues to have poor appetite, fevers, abdominal pain, distention, and loose stools. His work-up should include U/S and/or CT to evaluate for deep SSI. He is already 6 days post-op so imaging is indicated at this time.

Clinical Pearls

- There are no early signs (within 48 hours) of symptoms that reliably predict the development of an abdominal or pelvic abscess.
- Tolerating a regular diet on postoperative day 3 appears to be a good negative predictor for deep space infection.
- Diagnostic imaging of the abdomen and pelvis before postoperative day 5 may overestimate the incidence of abscesses: fluid collections without a well-defined rind may still resolve with antibiotics and conservative measures alone.

References

1. van Rossem CC, Bolmers MD, Schreinemacher MH, van Geloven AA, Bemelman WA, Snapshot Appendicitis Collaborative Study G. Prospective nationwide outcome audit of surgery for suspected acute appendicitis. Br J Surg. 2016;103(1):144–51.
2. Tiboni S, Bhangu A, Hall NJ, Paediatric Surgery Trainees Research N, The National Surgical Research C. Outcome of appendicectomy in children performed in paediatric surgery units compared with general surgery units. Br J Surg. 2014;101(6):707–14.
3. Emil S, Laberge JM, Mikhail P, Baican L, Flageole H, Nguyen L, et al. Appendicitis in children: a ten-year update of therapeutic recommendations. J Pediatr Surg. 2003;38(2):236–42.

4. St Peter SD, Sharp SW, Holcomb GW 3rd, Ostlie DJ. An evidence-based definition for perforated appendicitis derived from a prospective randomized trial. J Pediatr Surg. 2008;43(12):2242–5.
5. Romano A, Parikh P, Byers P, Namias N. Simple acute appendicitis versus non-perforated gangrenous appendicitis: is there a difference in the rate of post-operative infectious complications? Surg Infect. 2014;15(5):517–20.
6. Almaramhy HH. Acute appendicitis in young children less than 5 years: review article. Ital J Pediatr. 2017;43(1):15.
7. Davenport M. Acute abdominal pain in children. BMJ. 1996;312(7029):498–501.
8. Irish MS, Pearl RH, Caty MG, Glick PL. The approach to common abdominal diagnosis in infants and children. Pediatr Clin N Am. 1998;45(4):729–72.
9. Dillman JR, Smith EA, Morani AC, Trout AT. Imaging of the pediatric peritoneum, mesentery and omentum. Pediatr Radiol. 2017;47(8):987–1000.
10. Alloo J, Gerstle T, Shilyansky J, Ein SH. Appendicitis in children less than 3 years of age: a 28-year review. Pediatr Surg Int. 2004;19(12):777–9.
11. Garey CL, Laituri CA, Little DC, Ostlie DJ, St Peter SD. Outcomes of perforated appendicitis in obese and nonobese children. J Pediatr Surg. 2011;46(12):2346–8.
12. Blanco FC, Sandler AD, Nadler EP. Increased incidence of perforated appendicitis in children with obesity. Clin Pediatr (Phila). 2012;51(10):928–32.
13. Kutasy B, Puri P. Appendicitis in obese children. Pediatr Surg Int. 2013;29(6):537–44.
14. Timmerman ME, Groen H, Heineman E, Broens PM. The influence of underweight and obesity on the diagnosis and treatment of appendicitis in children. Int J Color Dis. 2016;31(8):1467–73.
15. Tian Y, Sweeney JF, Wulkan ML, Heiss KF, Raval MV. The necessity of sociodemographic status adjustment in hospital value rankings for perforated appendicitis in children. Surgery. 2016;159(6):1572–82.
16. Putnam LR, Tsao K, Nguyen HT, Kellagher CM, Lally KP, Austin MT. The impact of socioeconomic status on appendiceal perforation in pediatric appendicitis. J Pediatr. 2016;170:156–60.e1.
17. Lassiter RL, Hatley RM. Differences in the management of perforated appendicitis in children by race and insurance status. Am Surg. 2017;83(9):996–1000.
18. Zwintscher NP, Steele SR, Martin MJ, Newton CR. The effect of race on outcomes for appendicitis in children: a nationwide analysis. Am J Surg. 2014;207(5):748–53; discussion 53.
19. Penfold RB, Chisolm DJ, Nwomeh BC, Kelleher KJ. Geographic disparities in the risk of perforated appendicitis among children in Ohio: 2001–2003. Int J Health Geogr. 2008;7:56.
20. Smink DS, Fishman SJ, Kleinman K, Finkelstein JA. Effects of race, insurance status, and hospital volume on perforated appendicitis in children. Pediatrics. 2005;115(4):920–5.
21. Buckius MT, McGrath B, Monk J, Grim R, Bell T, Ahuja V. Changing epidemiology of acute appendicitis in the United States: study period 1993–2008. J Surg Res. 2012;175(2):185–90.
22. Narsule CK, Kahle EJ, Kim DS, Anderson AC, Luks FI. Effect of delay in presentation on rate of perforation in children with appendicitis. Am J Emerg Med. 2011;29(8):890–3.
23. Bickell NA, Aufses AH Jr, Rojas M, Bodian C. How time affects the risk of rupture in appendicitis. J Am Coll Surg. 2006;202(3):401–6.
24. Frongia G, Mehrabi A, Ziebell L, Schenk JP, Gunther P. Predicting postoperative complications after pediatric perforated appendicitis. J Investig Surg. 2016;29(4):185–94.
25. Obayashi J, Ohyama K, Manabe S, Tanaka K, Nagae H, Shima H, et al. Are there reliable indicators predicting post-operative complications in acute appendicitis? Pediatr Surg Int. 2015;31(12):1189–93.
26. Serres SK, Cameron DB, Glass CC, Graham DA, Zurakowski D, Karki M, et al. Time to appendectomy and risk of complicated appendicitis and adverse outcomes in children. JAMA Pediatr. 2017;171(8):740–6.
27. Habre W, Disma N, Virag K, Becke K, Hansen TG, Johr M, et al. Incidence of severe critical events in paediatric anaesthesia (APRICOT): a prospective multicentre observational study in 261 hospitals in Europe. Lancet Respir Med. 2017;5(5):412–25.

28. Oncu M, Calik A, Alhan E. A comparison of the simple ligation and ligation inversion of the appendiceal stump after appendectomy. Chir Ital. 1991;43(5–6):206–10.
29. van Rossem CC, van Geloven AA, Schreinemacher MH, Bemelman WA, Snapshot Appendicitis Collaborative Study G. Endoloops or endostapler use in laparoscopic appendectomy for acute uncomplicated and complicated appendicitis: no difference in infectious complications. Surg Endosc. 2017;31(1):178–84.
30. Safavi A, Langer M, Skarsgard ED. Endoloop versus endostapler closure of the appendiceal stump in pediatric laparoscopic appendectomy. Can J Surg. 2012;55(1):37–40.
31. Horvath P, Lange J, Bachmann R, Struller F, Konigsrainer A, Zdichavsky M. Comparison of clinical outcome of laparoscopic versus open appendectomy for complicated appendicitis. Surg Endosc. 2017;31(1):199–205.
32. Oka T, Kurkchubasche AG, Bussey JG, Wesselhoeft CW Jr, Tracy TF Jr, Luks FI. Open and laparoscopic appendectomy are equally safe and acceptable in children. Surg Endosc. 2004;18(2):242–5.
33. Jaschinski T, Mosch C, Eikermann M, Neugebauer EA. Laparoscopic versus open appendectomy in patients with suspected appendicitis: a systematic review of meta-analyses of randomised controlled trials. BMC Gastroenterol. 2015;15:48.
34. Sauerland S, Jaschinski T, Neugebauer EA. Laparoscopic versus open surgery for suspected appendicitis. Cochrane Database Syst Rev. 2010;10:CD001546.
35. Nataraja RM, Teague WJ, Galea J, Moore L, Haddad MJ, Tsang T, et al. Comparison of intraabdominal abscess formation after laparoscopic and open appendicectomies in children. J Pediatr Surg. 2012;47(2):317–21.
36. Newman K, Ponsky T, Kittle K, Dyk L, Throop C, Gieseker K, et al. Appendicitis 2000: variability in practice, outcomes, and resource utilization at thirty pediatric hospitals. J Pediatr Surg. 2003;38(3):372–9; discussion 9.
37. Hajibandeh S, Hajibandeh S, Kelly A, Shah J, Khan RMA, Panda N, et al. Irrigation versus suction alone in laparoscopic appendectomy: is dilution the solution to pollution? A systematic review and meta-analysis. Surg Innov. 2018;25(2):174–82.
38. Snow HA, Choi JM, Cheng MW, Chan ST. Irrigation versus suction alone during laparoscopic appendectomy; a randomized controlled equivalence trial. Int J Surg. 2016;28:91–6.
39. St Peter SD, Adibe OO, Iqbal CW, Fike FB, Sharp SW, Juang D, et al. Irrigation versus suction alone during laparoscopic appendectomy for perforated appendicitis: a prospective randomized trial. Ann Surg. 2012;256(4):581–5.
40. St Peter SD, Snyder CL. Operative management of appendicitis. Semin Pediatr Surg. 2016;25(4):208–11.
41. Fraser JD, Aguayo P, Sharp SW, Snyder CL, Holcomb GW 3rd, Ostlie DJ, et al. Physiologic predictors of postoperative abscess in children with perforated appendicitis: subset analysis from a prospective randomized trial. Surgery. 2010;147(5):729–32.
42. Daskalakis K, Juhlin C, Pahlman L. The use of pre- or postoperative antibiotics in surgery for appendicitis: a systematic review. Scand J Surg. 2014;103(1):14–20.
43. Ali K, Latif H, Ahmad S. Frequency of wound infection in non-perforated appendicitis with use of single dose preoperative antibiotics. J Ayub Med Coll Abbottabad. 2015;27(2):378–80.
44. Skarda DE, Schall K, Rollins M, Andrews S, Olson J, Greene T, et al. Response-based therapy for ruptured appendicitis reduces resource utilization. J Pediatr Surg. 2014;49(12):1726–9.
45. Guillet-Caruba C, Cheikhelard A, Guillet M, Bille E, Descamps P, Yin L, et al. Bacteriologic epidemiology and empirical treatment of pediatric complicated appendicitis. Diagn Microbiol Infect Dis. 2011;69(4):376–81.
46. Chen CY, Chen YC, Pu HN, Tsai CH, Chen WT, Lin CH. Bacteriology of acute appendicitis and its implication for the use of prophylactic antibiotics. Surg Infect. 2012;13(6):383–90.
47. Bassrawi RK, Al-Otaibi FE. Perforated acute appendicitis complicated by multiple intraabdominal abscesses caused by Enterococcus Avium in a non-compromised child. Saudi Med J. 2009;30(9):1231–2.

48. Burnett RJ, Haverstock DC, Dellinger EP, Reinhart HH, Bohnen JM, Rotstein OD, et al. Definition of the role of enterococcus in intraabdominal infection: analysis of a prospective randomized trial. Surgery. 1995;118(4):716–21; discussion 21–3.

49. Lee SL, Islam S, Cassidy LD, Abdullah F, Arca MJ, American Pediatric Surgical Association O, et al. Antibiotics and appendicitis in the pediatric population: an American Pediatric Surgical Association Outcomes and Clinical Trials Committee systematic review. J Pediatr Surg. 2010;45(11):2181–5.

50. Fraser JD, Aguayo P, Leys CM, Keckler SJ, Newland JG, Sharp SW, et al. A complete course of intravenous antibiotics vs a combination of intravenous and oral antibiotics for perforated appendicitis in children: a prospective, randomized trial. J Pediatr Surg. 2010;45(6):1198–202.

51. Loux TJ, Falk GA, Burnweit CA, Ramos C, Knight C, Malvezzi L. Early transition to oral antibiotics for treatment of perforated appendicitis in pediatric patients: confirmation of the safety and efficacy of a growing national trend. J Pediatr Surg. 2016;51(6):903–7.

52. Kronman MP, Oron AP, Ross RK, Hersh AL, Newland JG, Goldin A, et al. Extended- versus narrower-spectrum antibiotics for appendicitis. Pediatrics. 2016;138(1):e20154547.

53. Dickinson CM, Coppersmith NA, Luks FI. Early predictors of abscess development after perforated pediatric appendicitis. Surg Infect. 2017;18(8):886–9.

54. Shimizu T, Ishizuka M, Kubota K. The preoperative serum C-reactive protein level is a useful predictor of surgical site infections in patients undergoing appendectomy. Surg Today. 2015;45(11):1404–10.

55. Gorter RR, van den Boom AL, Heij HA, Kneepkens CM, Hulsker CC, Tenhagen M, et al. A scoring system to predict the severity of appendicitis in children. J Surg Res. 2016;200(2):452–9.

56. Chen CL, Chao HC, Kong MS, Chen SY. Risk factors for prolonged hospitalization in pediatric appendicitis patients with medical treatment. Pediatr Neonatol. 2017;58(3):223–8.

57. Parra JA, Revuelta S, Gallego T, Bueno J, Berrio JI, Farinas MC. Prosthetic mesh used for inguinal and ventral hernia repair: normal appearance and complications in ultrasound and CT. Br J Radiol. 2004;77(915):261–5.

58. Pham XD, Sullins VF, Kim DY, Range B, Kaji AH, de Virgilio CM, et al. Factors predictive of complicated appendicitis in children. J Surg Res. 2016;206(1):62–6.

59. Zouari M, Abid I, Sallami S, Guitouni A, Ben Dhaou M, Jallouli M, et al. Predictive factors of complicated appendicitis in children. Am J Emerg Med. 2017;35(12):1982–3.

60. Bech-Larsen SJ, Lalla M, Thorup JM. The influence of age, duration of symptoms and duration of operation on outcome after appendicitis in children. Dan Med J. 2013;60(8):A4678.

61. Tanaka S, Ishihara K, Uenishi T, Hashiba R, Kurashima Y, Ohno K, et al. Management of postoperative intraabdominal abscess in laparoscopic versus open appendectomy. Osaka City Med J. 2013;59(1):1–7.

62. Nielsen JW, Kurtovic KJ, Kenney BD, Diefenbach KA. Postoperative timing of computed tomography scans for abscess in pediatric appendicitis. J Surg Res. 2016;200(1):1–7.

63. Young JY, Kim DS, Muratore CS, Kurkchubasche AG, Tracy TF Jr, Luks FI. High incidence of postoperative bowel obstruction in newborns and infants. J Pediatr Surg. 2007;42(6):962–5; discussion 5.

64. Ouaissi M, Gaujoux S, Veyrie N, Deneve E, Brigand C, Castel B, et al. Post-operative adhesions after digestive surgery: their incidence and prevention: review of the literature. J Visc Surg. 2012;149(2):e104–14.

65. Ellozy SH, Harris MT, Bauer JJ, Gorfine SR, Kreel I. Early postoperative small-bowel obstruction: a prospective evaluation in 242 consecutive abdominal operations. Dis Colon Rectum. 2002;45(9):1214–7.

66. De Wilde RL, Brolmann H, Koninckx PR, Lundorff P, Lower AM, Wattiez A, et al. Prevention of adhesions in gynaecological surgery: the 2012 European field guideline. Gynecol Surg. 2012;9(4):365–8.

67. Elraiyah T, Hashim Y, Elamin M, Erwin PJ, Zarroug AE. The effect of appendectomy in future tubal infertility and ectopic pregnancy: a systematic review and meta-analysis. J Surg Res. 2014;192(2):368–74.e1.

68. Hookman P, Barkin JS. *Clostridium difficile* associated infection, diarrhea and colitis. World J Gastroenterol. 2009;15(13):1554–80.
69. McConnie R, Kastl A. *Clostridium Difficile*, colitis, and colonoscopy: pediatric perspective. Curr Gastroenterol Rep. 2017;19(8):34.
70. Siribumrungwong B, Chantip A, Noorit P, Wilasrusmee C, Ungpinitpong W, Chotiya P, et al. Comparison of superficial surgical site infection between delayed primary versus primary wound closure in complicated appendicitis: a randomized controlled trial. Ann Surg. 2018;267(4):631–7.
71. Brasel KJ, Borgstrom DC, Weigelt JA. Cost-utility analysis of contaminated appendectomy wounds. J Am Coll Surg. 1997;184(1):23–30.
72. Duggan EM, Marshall AP, Weaver KL, St Peter SD, Tice J, Wang L, et al. A systematic review and individual patient data meta-analysis of published randomized clinical trials comparing early versus interval appendectomy for children with perforated appendicitis. Pediatr Surg Int. 2016;32(7):649–55.
73. Solomkin JS, Mazuski JE, Bradley JS, Rodvold KA, Goldstein EJ, Baron EJ, et al. Diagnosis and management of complicated intra-abdominal infection in adults and children: guidelines by the Surgical Infection Society and the Infectious Diseases Society of America. Surg Infect. 2010;11(1):79–109.
74. Gasior AC, Marty Knott E, Ostlie DJ, St Peter SD. To drain or not to drain: an analysis of abscess drains in the treatment of appendicitis with abscess. Pediatr Surg Int. 2013;29(5):455–8.
75. Siewert B, Tye G, Kruskal J, Sosna J, Opelka F, Raptopoulos V, et al. Impact of CT-guided drainage in the treatment of diverticular abscesses: size matters. AJR Am J Roentgenol. 2006;186(3):680–6.
76. Fagenholz PJ, Peev MP, Thabet A, Michailidou M, Chang Y, Mueller PR, et al. Abscess due to perforated appendicitis: factors associated with successful percutaneous drainage. Am J Surg. 2016;212(4):794–8.
77. Lasson A, Lundagards J, Loren I, Nilsson PE. Appendiceal abscesses: primary percutaneous drainage and selective interval appendicectomy. Eur J Surg. 2002;168(5):264–9.
78. Rajak CL, Gupta S, Jain S, Chawla Y, Gulati M, Suri S. Percutaneous treatment of liver abscesses: needle aspiration versus catheter drainage. AJR Am J Roentgenol. 1998;170(4):1035–9.
79. Holzheimer RG, Mannick JA, editors. Surgical treatment: evidence-based and problem-oriented. Munich: Zuckschwerdt; 2001.
80. Fowler GR II. Observations upon appendicitis. Ann Surg. 1894;19(2):146–71.
81. Fowler GRI. Reichel on etiology and treatment of acute peritonitis. Ann Surg. 1890;12(1):43–5.
82. McDaniel JD, Warren MT, Pence JC, Ey EH. Ultrasound-guided transrectal drainage of deep pelvic abscesses in children: a modified and simplified technique. Pediatr Radiol. 2015;45(3):435–8.
83. Chung T, Hoffer FA, Lund DP. Transrectal drainage of deep pelvic abscesses in children using a combined transrectal sonographic and fluoroscopic guidance. Pediatr Radiol. 1996;26(12):874–8.
84. Kimura T, Shibata M, Ohhara M. Effective laparoscopic drainage for intra-abdominal abscess not amenable to percutaneous approach: report of two cases. Dis Colon Rectum. 2005;48(2):397–9.
85. Clark JJ, Johnson SM. Laparoscopic drainage of intraabdominal abscess after appendectomy: an alternative to laparotomy in cases not amenable to percutaneous drainage. J Pediatr Surg. 2011;46(7):1385–9.
86. Esposito S, Umbrello G, Castellazzi L, Principi N. Treatment of *Clostridium difficile* infection in pediatric patients. Expert Rev Gastroenterol Hepatol. 2015;9(6):747–55.

Disparities in the Management of Appendicitis

14

Randi L. Lassiter and Robyn M. Hatley

Case Example

Imagine for a moment an 8-year-old boy with a 1-day history of diffuse abdominal pain which has since localized to his right lower quadrant. He is seen in a pediatric surgery clinic upon referral from his primary care physician. Now imagine a 9-year-old boy presenting to his local community emergency department with right lower quadrant abdominal pain for the past 12 hours, fever, and anorexia. Both children have appendicitis. Will they receive the same workup and treatment?

Introduction

Disparities are an unfortunate reality of healthcare delivery in the United States. What additional information about the children in the scenario presented above may influence their course? Perhaps their parents' education level and insurance status should not influence their care. While the evidence that these disparities exist is overwhelming, it should be noted that controversy about what constitutes best management of acute appendicitis complicates any discussion about disparities. Debates regarding ideal diagnostic and treatment algorithms have been discussed in the preceding chapters. We will review the literature on differences in disease severity upon

R. L. Lassiter
Department of Surgery, Medical College of Georgia at Augusta University, Augusta, GA, USA
e-mail: rlassiter@augusta.edu

R. M. Hatley (✉)
Department of Surgery, Medical College of Georgia at Augusta University, Augusta, GA, USA

Section of Pediatric Surgery, Children's Hospital of Georgia, Augusta, GA, USA
e-mail: rhatley@augusta.edu

© Springer Nature Switzerland AG 2019
C. J. Hunter (ed.), *Controversies in Pediatric Appendicitis*,
https://doi.org/10.1007/978-3-030-15006-8_14

presentation as well as differences in existing practice patterns and outcomes by age group, race, and socioeconomic status with an emphasis on healthcare delivery in North America. As the patient moves through the healthcare system from presentation to discharge, the decisions made at each step and the potential for delays influence the subsequent steps and overall patient outcome. We will see how patient characteristics can predict the timeliness and type of intervention for children like the ones presented above who have very similar disease processes. In the discussion, we propose potential solutions to minimize and address these disparities.

Presentation

Differences in disease severity among children based on demographic groups are present from the first point of contact with healthcare providers. Appendiceal perforation is largely considered to be the natural disease progression of untreated appendicitis. Perforated appendicitis is a more complex disease to treat and has a higher rate of complications. It has been established that younger children, those uninsured or underinsured, and minority children have a higher incidence of perforated appendicitis.

In a study of Washington state discharge data between 1987 and 1996, Bratton and colleagues demonstrated that children younger than age 5 had the highest risk of complicated appendicitis, defined by rupture, peritonitis, or abscess, with an adjusted odds ratio of 4.5. Furthermore, they found a 1.3-fold increase in complicated disease in children with Medicaid compared to children with private insurance [1]. A retrospective cohort study using national data from the 2000 Kids' Inpatient Database (KID), which includes over 32,000 cases of appendicitis, found disproportionately higher rates of perforated appendicitis among children younger than age 9, those from poorer zip codes, lacking private insurance, and minority children. Researchers found that children with minority race and ethnicity had a 36–40% higher odds of perforated appendicitis [2].

A single large institutional study was conducted at the Children's Memorial Hermann Hospital in Houston, Texas, to identify socioeconomic predictors of appendiceal perforation. The authors found an increased rate of perforation in communities with a lower household income, a lower proportion of adults with a college education, and a higher percentage of adults with less than a 12th grade education. Public insurance and younger age were found to be even stronger predictors of perforation than measures of socioeconomic status [3]. Within the Canadian system of universal healthcare in the Manitoba province, researchers found that lower rural socioeconomic status, northern area of residence, receiving care at the province's only pediatric tertiary care hospital, and younger age were positive predictors of appendiceal rupture [4]. While most of the data discussed to date have focused on North American disparities, similar disparities in the management of appendicitis are found internationally. Kong et al. demonstrated that rural patients in KwaZulu-Natal, South Africa, were more likely than urban patients to present with perforated appendicitis and four-quadrant intra-abdominal contamination. These patients were more likely to require open abdomen management and re-laparotomy for sepsis. The authors posited that rural patients' poorer outcomes could be due to difficulty and delays in reaching the regional hospital [5].

Using the Nationwide Inpatient Sample (NIS) and the Kids' Inpatient Database (KID), Kokoska and colleagues found that Black and Hispanic children were more likely to have complex or perforated appendicitis compared to Caucasians with odds ratios of 1.39 and 1.48, respectively [6]. Data pulled from the KID 6 years later demonstrated persistent and significant disparities in the rate of perforation at presentation such that 27.5% of Black children and 32.5% of Hispanic children presented with perforated disease compared to 23.9% of Caucasian children [7]. Livingston and Fairlie sought to quantify just how much of the racial disparities in perforation rates at presentation could be explained by differences in socioeconomic factors and insurance. They ultimately found that only a small amount of the gap in perforation rates (26.7% White, 35.5% Black, 36.5% Latino) could be attributed to income level. They calculated that income only accounted for 7.2% and 6.1% of the gap for Black and Latino children, respectively. Instead, a full two-thirds of the gap in perforation rates between White and Black patients could not be accounted for by any measurable factors [8].

It should be noted that delays in presentation do not correlate directly with perforation. Ladd et al. noted that Hispanic children had a higher rate of perforated appendicitis independent of delays in treatment, defined as the time for symptom onset to incision, whereas higher rates of perforation in Black children were likely due to delays in treatment [9]. The authors ultimately concluded that perforated appendicitis is a heterogeneous disease with a variable course determined by multiple factors. Their findings led them to propose that delay in treatment is a better metric for pediatric healthcare disparities than perforation rates. As we will see in the next section, disparate delays in treatment are not limited to time from symptom onset to hospital presentation. There are measurable differences in when and how children are treated once they reach the hospital.

Evaluation

In a study conducted using data from the 2006 to 2009 National Hospital Ambulatory Medical Care Survey, significant differences were noted in the management of pediatric abdominal pain by race and ethnicity. Johnson et al. found no racial or ethnic differences in documentation of pain score. However, adjusting for confounders, including age, gender, triage level, hospital type and location, income, and insurance level, they discovered that non-Hispanic Black children were much less likely than non-Hispanic White children to receive any analgesics, narcotic or otherwise, even in cases of severe pain. Hispanic and non-Hispanic Black patients were more likely to have longer lengths of stay in the emergency department despite lack of differences in the use of diagnostic procedures or hospital admission [10].

A separate study conducted using the National Hospital Ambulatory Medical Care Survey from 2003 to 2010 was limited to children in emergency departments with an actual diagnosis of appendicitis. The study was designed to evaluate racial disparities in the administration of narcotics. Goya et al. found that Black children with moderate pain were less likely to receive analgesia. While there was no difference in the rate of administration for severe pain in their multivariable model, Black children with severe pain scores received analgesia significantly less frequently than White patients. The authors interpreted their findings to mean there were differences in the threshold for treatment of pain between races [11].

Examination of emergency department visits to tertiary children's hospitals belonging to the Child Health Corporation of America found that minorities and low-income children with appendicitis were less likely to undergo imaging for their appendicitis, including ultrasound, computed tomography (CT), and magnetic resonance imaging (MRI). Race and socioeconomic status together appeared to have a synergistic effect such that patients with Black race and low income had an odds of CT imaging that was much lower than would be predicted by race or income alone [12].

Treatment

Once the diagnosis of appendicitis has been made, timely treatment is necessary to avoid worsening morbidity. Lee et al. found that hospital delays in surgical intervention for pediatric acute appendicitis are associated with negative outcomes. They discovered that surgical treatment delayed until hospital day two or beyond was associated with increased likelihood of undergoing a colectomy, small bowel resection, or small bowel laceration repair, and increased complications, length of stay, and total hospital charges [13]. Unfortunately, these hospital-level delays occur more frequently among children of lower socioeconomic status and minority race. Black and Hispanic children have significantly longer length of time from presentation to surgery regardless of whether they have simple or perforated appendicitis [6]. Wang et al. found that high-income White children were taken to surgery the fastest but that high-income Blacks had a slower time to surgery and discharge than low-income Whites [12].

The benefits of laparoscopy over open appendectomy have been clearly established. Notwithstanding slightly longer operative times, laparoscopic appendectomy has been shown to be feasible, safe, and efficacious with shorter lengths of stay and less wound complications than the open approach [14]. These results have been verified for both uncomplicated and perforated appendicitis [15]. Despite an overall increase in the odds of undergoing laparoscopic appendectomy over a decade, analysis of the Nationwide Inpatient Sample and Kids' Inpatient Database from 1998 to 2007 demonstrated that Black patients were 20% less likely to undergo laparoscopic appendectomy compared to Caucasians patients [16].

In 2009, national racial disparities in the use of laparoscopy to treat pediatric appendicitis persisted but were marginally improved as Black children had 0.839 odds of undergoing a laparoscopic procedure compared to Caucasian children [7]. Interestingly, Wang et al. found that Black, Hispanic, and low-income children with appendicitis were less likely to have surgery for appendicitis at all at any time point compared to White and high-income patients [12].

In our own study evaluating disparities in operative and non-operative treatment of appendicitis, we specifically focused on children with complicated disease. After adjusting for multiple confounders, we found Black race, self-pay status, and rural

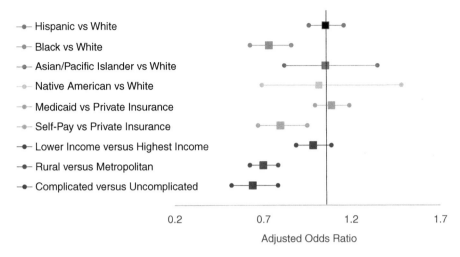

Fig. 14.1 Adjusted odds of undergoing laparoscopic appendectomy for perforated appendicitis. Multiple logistic regression was used to calculate the adjusted odds of undergoing laparoscopic appendectomy for children less than age 18 with perforated appendicitis. (Data is from the 2001 to 2010 National Inpatient Sample (NIS), the Healthcare Cost and Utilization Project (HCUP), and the Agency for Healthcare Research and Quality. Highest income is defined by patient zip code with a median income in the highest quartile. Metropolitan location was defined by a county with greater than 50,000 inhabitants, whereas a population of less than 50,000 people was defined as rural)

location to be independent predictors of undergoing open appendectomy (Fig. 14.1). Additionally, Black children admitted for perforated appendicitis were more likely not have an appendectomy and to undergo percutaneous drainage alone (Fig. 14.2). Hispanic children and those from rural communities were less likely to undergo percutaneous drainage alone compared to White children and those from metropolitan communities, respectively [17].

Sometimes the diagnosis of appendicitis is wrong, and non-incidental appendectomy is performed with removal of a normal appendix. This is the definition of a negative appendectomy. With the improvement of imaging technology, the rate of negative appendectomy is declining. By examining the Nationwide Inpatient Sample, Flum and Koepsell demonstrated that children less than age 5 are more likely to undergo negative appendectomy. They also found that negative appendectomy was associated with significantly longer length of stay, higher total hospital charges, and a higher rate of infectious complications [18]. Data from the California, Florida, and New York Inpatient Databases shows that White, female, and privately insured patients are more likely to undergo negative appendectomies. Negative appendectomies are associated with higher odds of complication, increased length of stay, and higher hospital costs than appendectomy performed for nonperforated appendicitis [19].

Outcomes

Socioeconomic status and race are ultimately predictors of outcome for pediatric appendicitis. There are measurable implications for delays in care and the differences in management discussed above. The downstream effects of disparities in access and treatment on the patients and their families include morbidity from complications, longer lengths of stay, and higher hospital charges.

Perforated appendicitis is associated with 97% higher hospital charges and 175% longer length of stay than non-perforated cases [2]. Kokoska et al. found that Black and Hispanic children had longer hospital stays and higher charges. While it makes sense that children with more complicated disease have longer lengths of stay, the authors also performed a subset analysis of children with simple appendicitis and still found that Black and Hispanic children had significantly longer lengths of stay and higher hospital charges [6]. Adjusting for perforation, Black and Hispanic children remain in the hospital for 0.76 days longer, and Hispanic patients are significantly more likely to have a complication [7]. Black children with appendicitis have a twofold higher risk of admission to an intensive care unit [12].

Same-day discharge is being used with increased frequency for cases of non-perforated appendicitis and also has variable application. When compared to Caucasians, Black and Hispanic children are less likely to undergo same-day discharge following appendectomy for non-perforated appendicitis. Of note, there are also regional differences such that hospitals in the south and midwest are less likely to utilize same-day discharge [20].

Potential Solutions

Multiple studies have shown improved outcomes for children with appendicitis when treated by subspecialty trained pediatric surgeons. In the hands of a pediatric surgeon, children with perforated appendicitis have lower complication rates and shorter

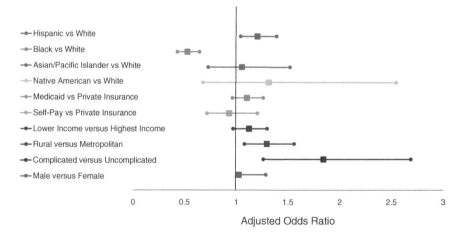

Fig. 14.2 Adjusted odds of undergoing surgery for perforated appendicitis. Multiple logistic regression was used to calculate the adjusted odds of undergoing surgery for children less than age 18 with perforated appendicitis. Surgery is defined as laparoscopic or open appendectomy, cecectomy, or partial colectomy. (Data is from the 2001 to 2010 National Inpatient Sample (NIS), the Healthcare Cost and Utilization Project (HCUP), and the Agency for Healthcare Research and Quality. Highest income is defined by patient zip code with a median income in the highest quartile. Metropolitan location was defined by a county with greater than 50,000 inhabitants, whereas a population of less than 50,000 people was defined as rural) Lassiter and Hatley [17]

lengths of stay than children treated by general surgeons [21]. Younger children, less than age 13, treated by pediatric surgeons have shorter lengths of stay and less hospital charges [22]. To date, most children receive their care at non-children's hospitals where there is an overall greater variation in resource utilization and outcomes than observed in children's hospitals. Children with perforated appendicitis treated at children's hospitals are more likely to undergo a laparoscopic appendectomy and have lower composite complication rates [23]. The natural question becomes whether racial and socioeconomic disparities are lessened by evaluation and treatment by pediatric surgeons at children's hospitals and/or teaching hospitals.

Kelley-Quon and colleagues studied differential patterns of pediatric perforated appendicitis depending on the hospital type within the state of California. They found that Hispanic children treated at children's hospitals actually had a higher rate of appendiceal perforation. While they did not find a difference in perforation rates by race within county hospitals, Black children treated at county hospitals had a higher rate of perforation compared with Black children treated at community hospitals [24]. In a multivariate analysis of a representative sample of national discharge data captured by the 1996–2002 Nationwide Inpatient Sample, White children overall were more likely to undergo laparoscopic appendectomy than Black children, but not other races. In contrast, at non-children's hospitals, Black, Hispanic, and Asian/Pacific Islander children had significantly lower odds of undergoing laparoscopic appendectomy compared to White children. At non-children's hospitals, children with private insurance were more likely to undergo laparoscopic appendectomy compared to those with Medicaid or Medicare. Thus racial and insurance-driven disparities were less pronounced at children's hospitals [25].

In a single institutional retrospective analysis of children treated for appendicitis at Children's Hospital in Columbus, Ohio, researchers noted a higher rate of perforation in children younger than age 6. Unlike previous studies examining national data, they did not find a significant difference in the rate of perforation or radiologic imaging studies by race, insurance status, income, or parental education level [26]. In another single-center study of 9424 patients evaluated in the Children's Hospital of Pittsburgh Emergency Department, Caperell et al. concluded that race and other demographic factors did not affect evaluation and management of acute abdominal pain, including imaging studies performed, therapy received, treatment with surgery, or final diagnosis. The most common etiology of abdominal pain in their population was constipation [27].

It is important to note that there is significant variability between children's hospitals which complicates the ability to generalize findings from a single institutional study to children's hospitals more broadly. A retrospective cohort study of children treated for appendicitis at free-standing children's hospitals demonstrated significant variation for a multitude of measures, including diagnostic imaging, laboratory testing, use of parenteral nutrition and peripherally inserted central catheter (PICC) lines, and median costs. They noted an impressive 4-fold difference in cost for uncomplicated disease and 4.6-fold difference for complicated disease [28]. Despite improved outcomes for appendicitis treated at children's hospitals, national data also reveals higher costs of care at children's hospitals and no difference in the length of stay between children's hospitals and non-children's hospitals [23]. Interestingly, another study of national discharge data captured by the Agency for Healthcare Research and Quality (AHRQ) Healthcare Cost and Utilization Project (HCUP) Kids' Inpatient Database (KID) demonstrated that hospitals with lower pediatric discharge volume had lower odds of ruptured appendicitis. There was no significant difference in the odds of appendiceal rupture when comparing teaching and nonteaching hospitals [2]. It also bears noting Black and Hispanic children are already more likely to present to children's hospitals than general community hospitals and are more likely to be treated at teaching hospitals than nonteaching hospitals [7].

In addition to concentrating care for pediatric appendicitis within institutions with specialized care, another proposed option to address socioeconomic disparities is to establish equal access to care. There are opportunities to learn about the impact of healthcare reform from the adult appendicitis literature. Loeher et al. conducted a retrospective cohort study of the odds of undergoing minimally invasive surgery in the state of Massachusetts compared to six control states. The authors found that following the 2006 healthcare reform, which expanded coverage for government-subsidized and uninsured individuals, Massachusetts saw a 3.71% increase in the probability of undergoing minimally invasive procedures for appendicitis and cholecystitis, effectively eliminating the disparity noted prior to the reform. Importantly, the authors found persistent disparity in the control states [29]. Upon examination of 11 Kaiser Permanente medical centers in Southern California, Lee et al. found persistent disparities despite equal access. Black and Hispanic adult patients were less likely to undergo laparoscopic appendectomy, while high- and middle-income patients were more likely to undergo laparoscopic appendectomy when compared to low-income patients [30]. In another study of the same database, the authors limited study to patients younger than age 18. They found no significant difference in perforation rates by race. They also found no significant difference in perforation by income or education level. Length of hospitalization was similar among all parental educational levels. However, Black children still had a longer length of stay, and higher income patients had a shorter length of stay compared to medium- and low-income families [31].

Discussion

Review of the literature reveals compelling disparities in the management of pediatric appendicitis. It is clear that pre-hospital access to care and severity of disease at presentation with perforated appendicitis hardly accounts for the multitude of differences in how children are managed after they reach the hospital. Both pre-hospital and intra-hospital delays have a real impact on outcome. Race, household income, and insurance status are independent predictors of how appendicitis will be managed, from when and where the child will present, whether and which surgery they will have, and what the child's ultimate outcome will be. The most at-risk groups for negative outcomes include children with minority race, lack of private insurance, and low-income households. In some cases, overly aggressive treatment for patients with majority race and higher socioeconomic status leads to worse outcomes including more radiation exposure from CT scans and a greater incidence of negative appendectomy.

As noted above, equivalent insurance and treatment at children's hospitals both lessen observed racial and socioeconomic disparities in the management of pediatric appendicitis without eliminating them. It is possible that some of the observed racial disparities in hospital charges may be partially driven by the fact that minority children are already more likely to receive their care in children's hospitals. It is our opinion that healthcare disparities represent opportunities for improvement. The first step to address disparities is to acknowledge their existence. Current and future generations of healthcare providers should be educated about existing disparities. While the abundance of literature suggests increased awareness of healthcare disparities, few, if any, studies have investigated whether knowledge of one's own implicit bias or varied practice patterns has any measurable effect on disparities at an individual or institutional level.

An additional way to address disparities may be to financially incentivize their elimination. Disparity at the hospital level can be a measurable quality metric much like catheter-associated urinary tract infections or central line-associated bloodstream infections. We propose that tying hospital-level disparities to reimbursement would inspire a culture of protocolized healthcare delivery. It would also incite interest on the behalf of administrators and clinicians to better understand the underlying causes of healthcare disparities and develop novel solutions which are unique to their patient population. Knott et al. found that instituting a clinical pathway for perforated appendicitis resulted in decreased time to advancement to a regular diet and shortened length of stay by more than 1 day while also decreasing the use of nasogastric tubes, PICCs, total parenteral nutrition, number of intravenous antibiotics, and laboratory draws [32]. We agree with Cameron and Rangel that there is a need to define meaningful variations in practice that result in poor resource utilization and result in worse outcomes, realizing that ideal practice patterns are dependent on resource availability and preferences of the patient population served. Not all variation or controversy is bad as it drives innovation [33].

Unfortunately, the demographic characteristics of children and their parents affect when and how appendicitis is managed. While this chapter focuses on appendicitis, given how common appendicitis is within the pediatric population, this disease process has the potential to serve as a barometer for overall disparities in the management of pediatric surgical emergencies. We are hopeful that these disparities can be eliminated. Addressing these disparities will require their acknowledgment as well as innovation and concerted investment to eradicate them.

Clinical Pearls

- Health disparities exist in the management and outcomes of children with appendicitis.
- Protocolized care and timely intervention may be a strategy to minimize unwanted outcomes in minority populations.

References

 1. Bratton SL, Haberkern CM, Waldhausen JH. Acute appendicitis risks of complications: age and Medicaid insurance. Pediatrics. 2000;106(1 Pt 1):75–8.
 2. Jablonski KA, Guagliardo MF. Pediatric appendicitis rupture rate: a national indicator of disparities in healthcare access. Popul Health Metrics. 2005;3(1):4.
 3. Putnam LR, Tsao K, Nguyen HT, Kellagher CM, Lally KP, Austin MT. The impact of socioeconomic status on appendiceal perforation in pediatric appendicitis. J Pediatr. 2016;170:156–60.
 4. Bratu I, Martens PJ, Leslie WD, Dik N, Chateau D, Katz A. Pediatric appendicitis rupture rate: disparities despite universal health care. J Pediatr Surg. 2008;43(11):1964–9.
 5. Kong VY, Van der Linde S, Aldous C, Handley JJ, Clarke DL. Quantifying the disparity in outcome between urban and rural patients with acute appendicitis in South Africa. S Afr Med J. 2013;103(10):742–5.
 6. Kokoska ER, Bird TM, Robbins JM, Smith SD, Corsi JM, Campbell BT. Racial disparities in the management of pediatric appendicitis. J Surg Res. 2007;137(1):83–8.
 7. Zwintscher NP, Steele SR, Martin MJ, Newton CR. The effect of race on outcomes for appendicitis in children: a nationwide analysis. Am J Surg. 2014;207(5):748–53; discussion 753.
 8. Livingston EH, Fairlie RW. Little effect of insurance status or socioeconomic condition on disparities in minority appendicitis perforation rates. Arch Surg. 2012;147(1):11–7.
 9. Ladd MR, Pajewski NM, Becher RD, Swanson JM, Gallaher JR, Pranikoff T, Neff LP. Delays in treatment of pediatric appendicitis: a more accurate variable for measuring pediatric healthcare inequalities? Am Surg. 2013;79(9):875–81.
10. Johnson TJ, Weaver MD, Borrero S, Davis EM, Myaskovsky L, Zuckerbraun NS, Kraemer KL. Association of race and ethnicity with management of abdominal pain in the emergency department. Pediatrics. 2013;132(4):e851–8.
11. Goyal MK, Kuppermann N, Cleary SD, Teach SJ, Chamberlain JM. Racial disparities in pain management of children with appendicitis in emergency departments. JAMA Pediatr. 2015;169(11):996–1002.
12. Wang L, Haberland C, Thurm C, Bhattacharya J, Park KT. Health outcomes in US children with abdominal pain at major emergency departments associated with race and socioeconomic status. PLoS One. 2015;10(8):e0132758.
13. Lee J, Tashjian DB, Moriarty KP. Missed opportunities in the treatment of pediatric appendicitis. Pediatr Surg Int. 2012;28(7):697–701.
14. Taqi E, Al Hadher S, Ryckman J, Su W, Aspirot A, Puligandla P, Flageole H, Laberge JM. Outcome of laparoscopic appendectomy for perforated appendicitis in children. J Pediatr Surg. 2008;43(5):893–5.
15. Wang X, Zhang W, Yang X, Shao J, Zhou X, Yuan J. Complicated appendicitis in children: is laparoscopic appendectomy appropriate? A comparative study with the open appendectomy – our experience. J Pediatr Surg. 2009;44(10):1924–7.
16. Oyetunji TA, Nwomeh BC, Ong'uti SK, Gonzalez DO, Cornwell EE 3rd, Fullum TM. Laparoscopic appendectomy in children with complicated appendicitis: ethnic disparity amid changing trend. J Surg Res. 2011;170(1):e99–103.
17. Lassiter RL, Hatley RM. Differences in the management of perforated appendicitis in children by race and insurance status. Am Surg. 2017;83(9):996–1000.
18. Flum DR, Koepsell T. The clinical and economic correlates of misdiagnosed appendicitis: nationwide analysis. Arch Surg. 2002;137(7):799–804; discussion 804.
19. Dubrovsky G, Rouch J, Huynh N, Friedlander S, Lu Y, Lee SL. Clinical and socioeconomic factors associated with negative pediatric appendicitis. J Surg Res. 2017;218:322–8.
20. Oyetunji TA, Gonzalez DO, Aguayo P, Nwomeh BC. Variability in same-day discharge for pediatric appendicitis. J Surg Res. 2015;199(1):159–63.
21. Alexander F, Magnuson D, DiFiore J, Jirousek K, Secic M. Specialty versus generalist care of children with appendicitis: an outcome comparison. J Pediatr Surg. 2001;36(10):1510–3.

22. Kokoska ER, Minkes RK, Silen ML, Langer JC, Tracy TF Jr, Snyder CL, Dillon PA, Weber TR. Effect of pediatric surgical practice on the treatment of children with appendicitis. Pediatrics. 2001;107(6):1298–301.
23. Tian Y, Heiss KF, Wulkan ML, Raval MV. Assessment of variation in care and outcomes for pediatric appendicitis at children's and non-children's hospitals. J Pediatr Surg. 2015;50(11):1885–92.
24. Kelley-Quon LI, Tseng CH, Jen HC, Lee SL, Shew SB. Hospital type as a metric for racial disparities in pediatric appendicitis. J Am Coll Surg. 2013;216(1):74–82.
25. Hagendorf BA, Liao JG, Price MR, Burd RS. Evaluation of race and insurance status as predictors of undergoing laparoscopic appendectomy in children. Ann Surg. 2007;245(1):118–25.
26. Nwomeh BC, Chisolm DJ, Caniano DA, Kelleher KJ. Racial and socioeconomic disparity in perforated appendicitis among children: where is the problem? Pediatrics. 2006;117(3):870–5.
27. Caperell K, Pitetti R, Cross KP. Race and acute abdominal pain in a pediatric emergency department. Pediatrics. 2013;131(6):1098–106.
28. Rice-Townsend S, Barnes JN, Hall M, Baxter JL, Rangel SJ. Variation in practice and resource utilization associated with the diagnosis and management of appendicitis at freestanding children's hospitals: implications for value-based comparative analysis. Ann Surg. 2014;259(6):1228–34.
29. Loehrer AP, Song Z, Auchincloss HG, Hutter MM. Massachusetts health care reform and reduced racial disparities in minimally invasive surgery. JAMA Surg. 2013;148(12):1116–22.
30. Lee SL, Yaghoubian A, Stark R, Shekherdimian S. Equal access to healthcare does not eliminate disparities in the management of adults with appendicitis. J Surg Res. 2011;170(2):209–13.
31. Lee SL, Shekherdimian S, Chiu VY. Comparison of pediatric appendicitis outcomes between teaching and nonteaching hospitals. J Pediatr Surg. 2010;45(5):894–7.
32. Knott EM, Gasior AC, Ostlie DJ, Holcomb GW 3rd, St Peter SD. Decreased resource utilization since initiation of institutional clinical pathway for care of children with perforated appendicitis. J Pediatr Surg. 2013;48(6):1395–8.
33. Cameron DB, Rangel SJ. Variation in pediatric surgical care. Semin Pediatr Surg. 2015;24(6):291–4.

Appendicitis: Unusual Complications and Outcomes

15

John Aiken

Introduction

Children with uncomplicated appendicitis who undergo prompt laparoscopic appendectomy have a low incidence of complications (1–3%) and typically make rapid recovery to full wellness and return to normal activities [1]. In contrast, children with complicated or perforated appendicitis are at risk for substantial morbidity, long hospital stays, and have an adverse event rate of 15–40%. The morbidity in association with complicated appendicitis has generated robust inquiry, debate, and controversy as to best approach to improve outcomes.

Primary outcome measures in pediatric appendicitis include overall complication rate, incidence of surgical site infections and intra-abdominal abscess, postoperative bowel obstruction, incisional hernia, and fecal fistula.

Secondary outcome measures include length of hospital stay, readmission rate, time to return to full activities, treatment-related costs, resource utilization, quality of life, and parent and patient satisfaction scores.

Intraoperative Complications

The surgical management of acute appendicitis has been the standard of care for more than a century. In earlier times, without antibiotics and when all surgery was "open", surgical complications were common in acute appendicitis. In current practice, with advanced laparoscopic techniques, intraoperative technical complications are rare.

J. Aiken (✉)
Children's Hospital of Wisconsin, Milwaukee, WI, USA

Medical College of Wisconsin, Wauwatosa, WI, USA
e-mail: JAiken@chw.org

© Springer Nature Switzerland AG 2019
C. J. Hunter (ed.), *Controversies in Pediatric Appendicitis*,
https://doi.org/10.1007/978-3-030-15006-8_15

Bleeding may occur with failure to secure the appendiceal artery during dissection or inadvertent injury to the intestinal mesentery. Iatrogenic bowel injury or injury to adherent structures, while uncommon, can occur during dissection to mobilize the appendix or to identify the base in the setting of a dense inflammatory reaction. Direct injury to adjacent bowel is most often only serosal, rarely full-thickness bowel injury. The bladder and the fallopian tube in girls may, on rare occasion, be injured by direct manipulation or thermal injury from the electrocautery. All of these complications are generally easily managed when promptly recognized with minimal morbidity [2].

Laparoscopic Appendectomy

In the open appendectomy era, operative exploration, particularly in complicated or perforated appendicitis, was wrought with an intimidating degree of complications and morbidity: large incisions, high rates of wound infection and postoperative intra-abdominal abscesses, fascial dehiscence, bleeding, abdominal injuries to friable bowel or adjacent structures, and prolonged ileus and antibiotics postoperatively. Drains, central lines, and parenteral nutrition were commonplace; morbidity was substantial.

The clear emergence of the laparoscopic approach for appendectomy on numerous studies and meta-analyses as superior to open appendectomy on essentially all metrics has significantly reduced complications and improved outcomes: decreased risk of wound infection, decreased pain and use of analgesic medications, decreased hospital stay, reduced postoperative ileus, improved cosmesis, and faster return to normal activities. The Pediatric Health Information System database shows the laparoscopic approach is now used in >90% of appendectomies, both simple and complicated. During the early experience with laparoscopy for perforated appendicitis, some authors reported longer operative times and an increased incidence of postoperative intra-abdominal abscess nearly threefold compared to open appendectomy; however, more recent literature clearly confirms reduced operative times and no difference in abscess risk between the open and laparoscopic approach based on multiple prospective trials, meta-analyses, and large, multi-institutional comparative series [3].

The laparoscopic technique has increased risks in children compared to adults during trocar placement. Injury to the intestines, intra-abdominal viscera, or major blood vessels (aorta, iliac vessels, inferior vena cava) are all reported during trocar insertion, presumed related to laxity of the abdominal wall in children. These injuries may be more likely in obese children with a thickened abdominal wall leading to the need for excessive force to be applied during trocar insertion. The sequelae of abdominal wall vessel injury are generally minimal: pain and hematoma formation at the trocar site. Many pediatric surgeons prefer an open technique for trocar insertion at the umbilical site prior to insufflation for safety, particularly in young children and children with thin body habitus. Occasionally, device malfunction can contribute to these types of injuries.

The laparoscopic approach, with small incisions and protective trocars, significantly lowers the incidence of surgical site infections compared to open appendectomy [4]. Furthermore, the laparoscopic approach minimizes the morbidity of wound complications when they do occur, a perennial problem with open appendectomy. The administration of intravenous antibiotics once the diagnosis of acute appendicitis has been made or suspected and effective re-dosing at the time of surgery have been consistently shown to lower the incidence of superficial SSI in appendicitis. Cameron and colleagues recently used the PHIS and ACS-Pediatric NSQIP databases to investigate the use of extended spectrum (piperacillin/tazobactam) or narrow spectrum (cefoxitin or ceftriaxone and metronidazole) in uncomplicated (i.e., non-perforated) acute appendicitis. Costs of the different regimens were similar, and readmission rates and hospital revisits were similar between the matched groups. The surgical site infection rate was 1.8% overall with no difference for the extended versus the narrow spectrum antibiotics [5]. This may provide an opportunity for improved stewardship of the use of extended spectrum antibiotics in uncomplicated appendicitis.

Laparoscopic appendectomy has become the standard of care in children in acute uncomplicated appendicitis. It is generally a 30–60 minute operation with a low complication rate and excellent outcomes. The incidence of superficial surgical site infections (SSI) with laparoscopic appendectomy in uncomplicated appendicitis is 1%, and the incidence of postoperative intra-abdominal abscess is generally <1%. All other short- and long-term complications after laparoscopic appendectomy for uncomplicated appendicitis are exceedingly rare. Length of stay is generally 12–24 hours, and many pediatric centers now have clinical pathway guidelines that allow for same day discharge open appendectomy is reserved for selected cases based on preoperative assessment and imaging, such as marked abdominal distension, or when during the laparoscopic approach the procedure is deemed technically difficult or unsafe.

In contrast to simple appendicitis, complicated appendicitis (perforated appendicitis with peritonitis, appendicular inflammatory mass, and perforated appendicitis with well-defined abscess) is associated with a complication rate of 15–40%. Early complications include intra-abdominal abscess (20–30%), superficial SSI, and small bowel obstruction. Patient morbidity is high, and outcomes are challenged with a broad array of adverse events: increased length of hospital stay, need for postoperative CT scans, emergency room revisits, unplanned reoperations and interventional procedures (drains and PICC lines), use of parenteral nutrition, and significant delay in return to wellness and full activities. Hospital costs are doubled in complicated appendicitis, and nationwide the readmission rate is estimated at 12.8%.

Outcomes and Resource Utilization

Acute appendicitis is estimated to account for greater than one million pediatric hospital admission days per year and at a cost of >$680 million per year. Despite the frequency of appendicitis in children, the heterogeneity of the patients across age groups and severity of illness scale has been an obstacle to establishing standardized outcome measures. Optimal treatment remains elusive, particularly for complicated appendicitis, representing as much as one half the patients in many centers at presentation. Clinical management is characterized by marked variability in resource utilization, outcomes, and costs, both within children's hospitals and in the community [6, 7]. Variation in care has been identified as a key driver in healthcare costs and has been targeted for quality improvement efforts to steward resource utilization and improve outcomes [8].

Recent research efforts have sought to identify the influence of surgeon experience (operative volume, specialty training) and hospital factors (hospital designation) on outcomes in children with surgical illness [9, 10]. The American College of Surgeons has recently instituted a children's hospital verification designation program to optimize the surgical care of children. Numerous studies have demonstrated improved outcomes in acute appendicitis treated in specialty children's centers by fellowship-trained pediatric surgeons and other pediatric specialists, particularly in younger children [11].

Operative volume, fellowship-trained pediatric surgeons, pediatric anesthetists, and established evidence-based clinical pathways are likely critical drivers of these improved outcomes [12]. Despite these existing data, the 2012 report from the KIDS national database, a retrospective review found that 82.4% of patients ages 2–18 years who underwent appendectomy were treated at a non-children's hospitals. In hospitalizations for patients identified as having perforated appendicitis, the mean case volume per hospital was 7, and the median case volume per hospital was 2 [13]. These volumes are undoubtedly low.

Another area of controversy is drainage procedures for intra-abdominal abscesses [14]. Drainage procedures for intra-abdominal abscess by interventional radiology have their own potential complications and have been consistently identified as a major factor in increased length of stay and escalation of hospital costs in acute appendicitis. Risks associated with percutaneous drainage of intra-abdominal abscesses are reported in 2–3% of percutaneous drain procedures and include bleeding, intestinal perforation, bladder perforation, fecal fistula formation, soft tissue abscess (buttock/thigh), and post procedure sepsis. While the number of complications is not high, the hospital course and time to recovery are often significantly impacted [15]. In addition, current reviews and meta-analyses demonstrate patients with drains consistently have increased use of CT scans contributing to the cumulative lifetime radiation risk. A more selective approach to antibiotic-alone management of smaller, asymptomatic abscesses and clinical practice guidelines to limit postoperative CT imaging before postoperative day 7 and directed by clinical criteria is likely to substantially reduce hospital costs, resource utilization, and radiation exposure without compromise of quality or safety measures [16].

Postoperative Intestinal Obstruction

Postoperative bowel obstruction and ileus are uncommon after uncomplicated appendicitis treated by laparoscopic appendectomy. The risk of bowel obstruction requiring reoperation is consistently reported around 0.7% in numerous large national database studies [17]. The risk is expectedly higher in open appendectomy and in patients with complicated or perforated appendicitis, historically reported from 0.5% to 10.7% in reviews with long-term follow-up. The laparoscopic approach is estimated to have as much as a fourfold decrease in the incidence of adhesive formation compared to open surgery. While adhesive postoperative bowel obstruction can occur as early as the first week postoperatively, the majority of cases occur following initial discharge in the first 1–2 years [18].

Unusual Pathology

Albeit rare, appendiceal carcinoid tumors are discovered incidentally in approximately 0.2% of children [19]. Typically these are small tumors with a low risk of lymphovascular invasion or extension. The rare occurrence of this finding may be cited in support of interval appendectomy following presumed perforated appendicitis, to prevent missing this diagnosis. In addition to rare tumor diagnoses, unusual infections may mimic appendicitis. For example, the pathologist may identify a parasite such as *Enterobius vermicularis* (pin worm) within the lumen of the appendix masquerading as appendicitis [20].

Rare Complications in Appendicitis

Fecal Fistula

Fecal fistula is a rare complication in appendicitis, occurring in <1% of patients. This may occur as sequelae of intra-abdominal infection/abscess in patients with complicated appendicitis or as a procedure-related complication of percutaneous drainage of an intra-abdominal abscess. Similar to intestinal fistulae seen in other surgical settings, fecal fistula in the setting of appendicitis will most often close spontaneously (>90%) with non-operative management provided coexisting disease is absent including foreign body, immune deficiency, malnutrition, and distal bowel obstruction. An important consideration in a patient with fecal fistula is the possibility of incipient Crohn's disease.

Long-Term Complications

Inflammatory Bowel Disease

The precise role of the appendix as part of the digestive tract remains unclear; however, some authors have suggested the appendix may have an immunological role. The appendix contains the highest amount of gut-associated lymphoid tissue (GALT) in the intestinal tract, and removal of the appendix may alter the intestinal tract bacterial microbiome. This finding has led to numerous studies investigating the possibility that removal of the appendix could have a role in the development of inflammatory bowel disease or cancer [21].

The incidence of Crohn's disease seems to be slightly higher after appendectomy [22]. Studies reporting on Crohn's disease demonstrated a median prevalence of 0.20% in patients who underwent appendectomy and 0.12% in study group controls. One study reported 2.3 times as many cases of Crohn's disease in the appendectomy group compared to the control group. Alternatively, it is also suggested that the higher prevalence of Crohn's disease, especially cases identified in early follow-up after appendectomy, might be related to the difficulties in diagnosing an incipient Crohn's disease [23, 24].

The incidence of ulcerative colitis is not changed after appendectomy. The mean prevalence of ulcerative colitis, reviewed in only a few studies, was 0.15% in patients after appendectomy and 0.19% in the studied controls. Andersson et al. actually reported a reduced risk of ulcerative colitis after appendectomy in patients <20 years of age, and this has been in other case-control studies [25].

Perforated Appendicitis and Subsequent Infertility in Girls

Although perforated appendicitis has been considered a risk factor for tubal infertility in women, epidemiologic evidence supporting this relation is inconsistent. Earlier reports of an increase in tubal infertility after appendectomy had significant limitations: study patients were adult women who had undergone appendectomy for perforated appendicitis in adult life; case numbers were small, and detailed investigations of infertility were lacking. In one study suggesting increased infertility in women after perforated appendicitis, critical analysis revealed that 20% of the patients reported with primary infertility had a history of pelvic inflammatory disease compared with only 3% of patients in the control group. A 2001 study investigating risk factors for tubal infertility in 121 women attending in vitro fertilization clinics in Toronto, Canada, found that history of acute appendicitis or perforated appendicitis was not a statistically significant risk factor for tubal infertility in their patients [26].

There are minimal reports in the literature that have specifically investigated infertility in women who had undergone appendectomy in childhood. Recently, a large cohort study from Sweden investigated fertility patterns in women (9840 patients over a 20-year period) who had undergone appendectomy when aged <15 years and demonstrated similar rates of first birth and distribution of parity between women with history of perforated appendicitis and control women. Women with a history of perforated appendicitis had a similar rate of first births as the control women and a similar distribution of parity at the end of follow-up (mean age 31.6 years) [27].

In another recent systematic review and meta-analysis, including electronic databases from inception until 2013, no statistically significant association was found between appendectomy and infertility; however, appendectomy was associated with a significantly increased risk of ectopic pregnancy [28].

In summary, these data indicate that perforated appendicitis before puberty does not appear to have long-term negative effects on female fertility. These data have important implications for clinical practice for counseling patients and families when young women present acutely with suspected acute appendicitis to refute a widely accepted approach that females should be considered for earlier surgery with a higher negative appendectomy rate to avoid perforation of the appendix and the concerns for future infertility.

Portal or Splenic Vein Thrombosis

Also exceedingly rare in the pediatric literature is the occurrence of superior mesenteric vein, portal vein, or splenic vein thrombosis in association with appendicitis [29]. The diagnosis tends to be delayed due its nonspecific symptoms. The condition can occur at presentation, in a patient with history suggestive of appendicitis that went unrecognized or after appendectomy in complicated appendicitis. This condition, termed pylephlebitis, is presumed a consequence of a convergence of factors: intra-abdominal infection and local sepsis producing a hypercoagulable state, dehydration, and bacterial invasion into the mesenteric venous system [30]. While exceptionally rare in children, the condition can be fatal if left undiagnosed or untreated. Presenting signs and symptoms are typically nonspecific: fevers, vague abdominal pain, poor appetite, weight loss, sweats, chills, malaise, and occasionally diarrhea. If thrombosis of the portal venous system occurs, patients may demonstrate signs and symptoms of portal hypertension. Affected patients frequently have elevated serum inflammatory markers (CRP, ESR) and blood cultures positive for enteric organisms: *Escherichia coli*, *Bacteroides fragilis*, *Proteus mirabilis*, *Klebsiella pneumoniae*, and *Enterobacter species*.

Diagnosis is made by ultrasound or CT demonstrating thrombus formation in the portomesenteric venous system and may extend into the splenic vein. A 1–2-week course of broad-spectrum antibiotics targeting gram-negative enteric bacteria and anaerobes is foundational therapy, and therapeutic anticoagulation is indicated to limit extension of the thrombus and to enhance natural fibrinolysis. In patients when the mesenteric thrombus occurs acutely, catheter-directed thrombolysis by interventional radiology is an option. Anticoagulation therapy is generally continued for 3–6 months, although patients may show almost complete resolution of thrombus as early as the first month of treatment. Liver abscess can also occur. The patient typically demonstrates a large, tender liver. Treatment is aspiration and antibiotics.

"Stump" Appendicitis

Incomplete removal of the appendix places a patient at risk for recurrent appendicitis, termed "stump" appendicitis. This is a rare event, and most surgeons will likely see only a few cases in a career. The time to occurrence is generally years after the initial surgery; however, occasionally stump appendicitis may occur even within the first year. Patients typically present with clinical signs and symptoms of acute appendicitis, and a definitive diagnosis is made with abdominal CT scan. Stump appendicitis has been reported after both laparoscopic and open appendectomy. It appears to be more likely after complicated appendicitis. It may be related to an incomplete appendectomy, leaving a small "stump" of appendix in place at the time of removal. The diagnosis of "stump" appendicitis is associated with significant morbidity as patients who developed stump appendicitis were more likely on the second surgery to have complicated appendicitis, have an open procedure, and undergo colectomy in surgical management.

Incisional or Port Site Hernia

The incidence of port site hernia following laparoscopy in adults is reported as 0.1–3%. In a recent systematic review, which included 37 studies, only four studies reported on the incidence of incisional hernia. The overall prevalence of incisional hernia was 0.7%. The vast majority of incisional hernias reported occurred in laparoscopic converted to open appendectomies. The data in children is expectedly sparse, and the incidence is likely underappreciated as many port site hernias would be asymptomatic and unrecognized. Limited studies suggest the incidence of port site hernia is higher in younger children, particularly children preschool age and younger. While risk factors for development of port site or incisional hernia in adults include infection, obesity, and diabetes, no risk factors have reliably been identified in children. Closure of all port sites does not obviate port site hernia; however, fascial closure of openings 10 mm or greater is performed by most pediatric surgeons.

Sarcopenia

Sarcopenia is defined as a decrease in skeletal muscle mass and has been shown to be associated with longer postoperative recovery and an increased risk of complications in adult surgical patients. Children with delayed presentation and complicated appendicitis may experience, in the course of illness, treatment, and recovery, an extended period of inadequate nutrition and be at risk for sarcopenia and potential worse outcomes. A particular risk identified in patients with sarcopenia appears to be a higher risk of poor wound healing and postoperative surgical site infections. In a recent retrospective review from Nationwide Children's Hospital in pediatric patients, nutritional assessment in select patients as part of preoperative risk assessment may provide important information that could identify patients who would benefit from early nutritional intervention and thereby potentially lower the incidence of complications and improve outcomes [31].

Conclusion

Complications in the management of appendicitis are low; however there are a few rare complications or outcomes that merit consideration especially when the postmanagement course follows an unexpected path. To minimize general complications and improve outcomes, it appears that management may best be performed by specialized providers in a high-volume center. This is especially true for the youngest patients.

Clinical Pearls

- Outcomes may be optimized by having specialized providers care for patients, and this is especially true for the younger patients.
- It appears unlikely that appendicitis significantly affects long-term fertility.
- Knowledge of rare outcomes and associations with appendicitis merit consideration when a patient has an unexpected postoperative course.

References

1. Rasmussen T, Fonnes S, Rosenberg J. Long-term complications of appendectomy: a systematic review. Scand J Surg. 2018;107(3):189–96.
2. Linnaus ME, Ostlie DJ. Complications in common general pediatric surgery procedures. Semin Pediatr Surg. 2016;25(6):404–11.
3. Andersson RE. Short and long-term mortality after appendectomy in Sweden 1987 to 2006. Influence of appendectomy diagnosis, sex, age, co-morbidity, surgical method, hospital volume, and time period. A national population-based cohort study. World J Surg. 2013;37(5):974–81.
4. Khiria LS, Ardhnari R, Mohan N, Kumar P, Nambiar R. Laparoscopic appendicectomy for complicated appendicitis: is it safe and justified?: a retrospective analysis. Surg Laparosc Endosc Percutan Tech. 2011;21(3):142–5.
5. Cameron DB, Melvin P, Graham DA, Glass CC, Serres SK, Kronman MP, et al. Extended versus narrow-spectrum antibiotics in the management of uncomplicated appendicitis in children: a propensity-matched comparative effectiveness study. Ann Surg. 2018;268(1):186–92.
6. Collins HL, Almond SL, Thompson B, Lacy D, Greaney M, Baillie CT, et al. Comparison of childhood appendicitis management in the regional paediatric surgery unit and the district general hospital. J Pediatr Surg. 2010;45(2):300–2.
7. Oyetunji TA, Ong'uti SK, Bolorunduro OB, Cornwell EE 3rd, Nwomeh BC. Pediatric negative appendectomy rate: trend, predictors, and differentials. J Surg Res. 2012;173(1):16–20.
8. Tian Y, Heiss KF, Wulkan ML, Raval MV. Assessment of variation in care and outcomes for pediatric appendicitis at children's and non-children's hospitals. J Pediatr Surg. 2015;50(11):1885–92.
9. Emil SG, Taylor MB. Appendicitis in children treated by pediatric versus general surgeons. J Am Coll Surg. 2007;204(1):34–9.
10. Somme S, To T, Langer JC. Effect of subspecialty training on outcome after pediatric appendectomy. J Pediatr Surg. 2007;42(1):221–6.
11. Kokoska ER, Minkes RK, Silen ML, Langer JC, Tracy TF Jr, Snyder CL, et al. Effect of pediatric surgical practice on the treatment of children with appendicitis. Pediatrics. 2001;107(6):1298–301.
12. McAteer JP, LaRiviere CA, Oldham KT, Goldin AB. Shifts towards pediatric specialists in the treatment of appendicitis and pyloric stenosis: trends and outcomes. J Pediatr Surg. 2014;49(1):123–7; discussion 7–8.
13. Masoomi H, Mills S, Dolich MO, Ketana N, Carmichael JC, Nguyen NT, et al. Comparison of outcomes of laparoscopic versus open appendectomy in children: data from the Nationwide Inpatient Sample (NIS), 2006–2008. World J Surg. 2012;36(3):573–8.
14. Keckler SJ, Tsao K, Sharp SW, Ostlie DJ, Holcomb GW 3rd, St Peter SD. Resource utilization and outcomes from percutaneous drainage and interval appendectomy for perforated appendicitis with abscess. J Pediatr Surg. 2008;43(6):977–80.

15. St Peter SD, Aguayo P, Fraser JD, Keckler SJ, Sharp SW, Leys CM, et al. Initial laparo-scopic appendectomy versus initial nonoperative management and interval appendectomy for perforated appendicitis with abscess: a prospective, randomized trial. J Pediatr Surg. 2010;45(1):236–40.
16. Williams RF, Interiano RB, Paton E, Eubanks JW, Huang EY, Langham MR, et al. Impact of a randomized clinical trial on children with perforated appendicitis. Surgery. 2014;156(2):462–6.
17. Tsao KJ, St Peter SD, Valusek PA, Keckler SJ, Sharp S, Holcomb GW 3rd, et al. Adhesive small bowel obstruction after appendectomy in children: comparison between the laparoscopic and open approach. J Pediatr Surg. 2007;42(6):939–42; discussion 42.
18. Kaselas C, Molinaro F, Lacreuse I, Becmeur F. Postoperative bowel obstruction after laparoscopic and open appendectomy in children: a 15-year experience. J Pediatr Surg. 2009;44(8):1581–5.
19. Fallon SC, Hicks MJ, Carpenter JL, Vasudevan SA, Nuchtern JG, Cass DL. Management of appendiceal carcinoid tumors in children. J Surg Res. 2015;198(2):384–7.
20. Zouari M, Louati H, Abid I, Trabelsi F, Ben Dhaou M, Jallouli M, et al. *Enterobius vermicularis*: a cause of abdominal pain mimicking acute appendicitis in children. A retrospective cohort study. Arch Iran Med. 2018;21(2):67–72.
21. Cakmak YO, Ergelen R, Ekinci G, Kaspar EC. The short appendix vermiformis as a risk factor for colorectal cancer. Clin Anat. 2014;27(3):498–502.
22. Andersson RE, Olaison G, Tysk C, Ekbom A. Appendectomy is followed by increased risk of Crohn's disease. Gastroenterology. 2003;124(1):40–6.
23. Kurina LM, Goldacre MJ, Yeates D, Seagroatt V. Appendicectomy, tonsillectomy, and inflammatory bowel disease: a case-control record linkage study. J Epidemiol Community Health. 2002;56(7):551–4.
24. Russel MG, Dorant E, Brummer RJ, van de Kruijs MA, Muris JW, Bergers JM, et al. Appendectomy and the risk of developing ulcerative colitis or Crohn's disease: results of a large case-control study. South Limburg Inflammatory Bowel Disease Study Group. Gastroenterology. 1997;113(2):377–82.
25. Andersson RE, Olaison G, Tysk C, Ekbom A. Appendectomy and protection against ulcerative colitis. N Engl J Med. 2001;344(11):808–14.
26. Urbach DR, Marrett LD, Kung R, Cohen MM. Association of perforation of the appendix with female tubal infertility. Am J Epidemiol. 2001;153(6):566–71.
27. Andersson R, Lambe M, Bergstrom R. Fertility patterns after appendicectomy: historical cohort study. BMJ. 1999;318(7189):963–7.
28. Elraiyah T, Hashim Y, Elamin M, Erwin PJ, Zarroug AE. The effect of appendectomy in future tubal infertility and ectopic pregnancy: a systematic review and meta-analysis. J Surg Res. 2014;192(2):368–74 e1.
29. Bakti N, Hussain A, El-Hasani S. A rare complication of acute appendicitis: superior mesenteric vein thrombosis. Int J Surg Case Rep. 2011;2(8):250–2.
30. Singal AK, Kamath PS, Tefferi A. Mesenteric venous thrombosis. Mayo Clin Proc. 2013;88(3):285–94.
31. Lopez JJ, Cooper JN, Albert B, Adler B, King D, Minneci PC. Sarcopenia in children with perforated appendicitis. J Surg Res. 2017;220:1–5.

Management of Acute Appendicitis in Special Pediatric Situations: Malignancy, Neutropenia, and Other Etiologies of Immune Suppression

16

Timothy B. Lautz

Case Example

A 5-year-old male on therapy for acute lymphoblastic leukemia presents with right lower quadrant abdominal pain. His absolute neutrophil count is $200/mm^3$. Diagnostic ultrasound reveals an enlarged (11 mm) appendix with periappendiceal fat stranding but no evidence of perforation. How should this child be managed?

Introduction

Given the relative frequency of both acute appendicitis and hematologic malignancies in children, it is inevitable that some children undergoing treatment for leukemia or lymphoma will develop acute appendicitis. Neutropenia is an unavoidable complication of treatment for these malignancies which creates a management dilemma for surgeons caring for these patients. On the one hand, laparoscopic appendectomy performed in the setting of neutropenia may increase the risk of surgical complications including wound dehiscence, appendiceal stump leak, and infectious complications. On the other hand, patients with neutropenia are at risk of major infectious complications, including sepsis, if appendicitis is inadequately treated.

Although neutropenia due to treatment for a hematologic malignancy is the most common cause of immune suppression confounding treatment for acute appendicitis, it is not the only etiology. A multitude of other diseases and disease treatments suppress the immune system and raise similar management concerns. Diseases affecting the immune system can be primary (e.g., severe combined immunodeficiency, common variable immunodeficiency, X-linked agammaglobulinemia) or

T. B. Lautz (✉)
Feinberg School of Medicine, Northwestern University, Chicago, IL, USA

Ann & Robert H. Lurie Children's Hospital of Chicago, Chicago, IL, USA
e-mail: TLautz@luriechildrens.org

© Springer Nature Switzerland AG 2019
C. J. Hunter (ed.), *Controversies in Pediatric Appendicitis*,
https://doi.org/10.1007/978-3-030-15006-8_16

secondary (e.g., acquired immunodeficiency syndrome). Other treatments associated with iatrogenic immunodeficiency include antineoplastic therapy, immunosuppression following transplant, and therapy for many immune and rheumatologic conditions.

Diagnosis of acute appendicitis in children with immune suppression may be confounded by masking of the typical presenting symptoms. Furthermore, even with modern imaging techniques, it can be difficult to differentiate appendicitis from neutropenic colitis ("typhlitis") which is almost always managed non-operatively. The presence of fever has been proposed as way to help distinguish "typhlitis" from appendicitis [1], but other authors have reported high rates of fever in neutropenic children with appendicitis [2].

While non-operative management of routine acute appendicitis has become an active area of study in recent years, much of the foundation for this approach came from experience managing patients with appendicitis in the setting of neutropenia. It has long been known that appendicitis can be successfully treated in the acute setting with antibiotic therapy, allowing for delayed removal of the appendix when the patient was better suited to undergo an operation.

This chapter will focus on the management of acute appendicitis in children with a known diagnosis of immune deficiency, particularly children with neutropenia secondary to antineoplastic therapy for malignancy. This is in contrast to the rare, but well-established, scenario where appendicitis is the initial presenting symptom for a hematologic malignancy due to lymphoid hyperplasia around the appendix.

Literature Review

Existing data on the management and outcome of children with acute appendicitis in the setting of immune suppression comes primarily from institutional case series of children with hematologic malignancies (Table 16.1). The largest series included 30 patients from 12 institutions in France [2]. Other reports have all included fewer than 15 patients. Two studies reported on the rate of appendicitis among their entire

Table 16.1 Case series of appendicitis management in children on therapy for malignancy

Study	# patients	% hematologic malignancy	% perforated	% early appendectomy[a]	Major complications
Chui [3]	10	70	40	100	3 deaths
Kim [4]	7	100[b]	57	100	None
Hobson [1]	7	100[b]	71	43	None
Mortellaro [5]	11	91	27	100	None
Scarpa [2]	30	90	27	20	3 laparotomies in delayed group
Singer [6]	5	80	0	100	None
Warad [7]	3	100[b]	33	100	1 abscess
Wiegering [8]	5	100[b]	20	0	None

[a]Within 2 days
[b]By study design

cohort of children undergoing therapy for hematologic malignancy, finding an incidence of 0.6–1.9% [1, 4, 7]. Patients with hematologic malignancy comprised >70% of the population in all reported studies.

The utilization of up-front surgery (within 2 days of diagnosis) varied from 0% to 100% in different series, averaging 56%. However, in the largest study, only 6 patients underwent up-front appendectomy, 17 had delayed appendectomy after a median of 32 days, and 7 patients had definitive non-operative treatment [2]. In another study, all five patients had successful non-operative treatment with meropenem monotherapy, although three had recurrent right lower quadrant symptoms managed with additional courses of antibiotic therapy [8].

The rate of perforated appendicitis varied from 0% to 71%, with a mean of 44%. Most studies reported no major operative morbidity or mortality. However in one study, three of ten children died in the postoperative period due to septicemia [3]. Major complications also occurred in two patients treated initially with antibiotic therapy who required emergent operation for life-threatening acute abdominal symptoms [2].

Data on children with appendicitis in the setting of other primary or secondary immune deficiencies is even more sparse. Of note, although the inflammatory infiltrate in acute appendicitis typically consists predominantly of neutrophils, children with congenital neutrophil deficiency can still develop appendicitis [9].

Administrative Data

Due to the paucity of existing data on the current management of appendicitis in children with neutropenia and appendicitis, a large, national administrative dataset was queried for further information. The Pediatric Health Information System (PHIS) database contains inpatient, emergency department, ambulatory surgery, and observation encounter-level data from over 49 not-for-profit, tertiary care pediatric hospitals in the United States.[1] For this study, data from 39 hospitals was included.

PHIS was queried from January 2013 through December 2017 for patients <18 years of age with a malignancy diagnosis admitted with concurrent diagnosis of acute appendicitis and chemotherapy-induced neutropenia or pancytopenia.[2]

---

[1] These hospitals are affiliated with the Children's Hospital Association (CHA) (Lenexa, KS). Data quality and reliability are assured through a joint effort between the CHA and participating hospitals. Portions of the data submission and data quality processes for the PHIS data set are managed by Truven Health Analytics (Ann Arbor, MI). For the purposes of external benchmarking, participating hospitals provide discharge/encounter data including demographics, diagnoses, and procedures. Nearly all of these hospitals also submit resource utilization data into PHIS. Data are de-identified at the time of data submission, and data are subjected to a number of reliability and validity checks before being included in the dataset.

[2] ICD-9 and ICD-10 codes

Acute appendicitis (K350, K352, K353, K3580, K3589, 540, 5400, 54009, 5401, or 5409).
Chemotherapy-induced neutropenia or pancytopenia (D701, D61810, 28411, or 28803).

Appendicitis with generalized peritonitis or peritoneal abscess was identified as "complicated."

During the study period, 116 children met inclusion criteria, including 64 boys (55.2%). Median age was 11 years (IQR 5–14). Seventy-four (63.8%) patients were white, and 44 (37.9%) were of Hispanic ethnicity. Fifty (43.1%) patients were admitted through the ED, while 29 (25.0%) had an initially elective admission. Forty-one patients (35.3%) spent time in the ICU during their admission. Ninety-four (81.0%) patients had a hematologic malignancy. Median length of stay was 21 days (IQR 9–45).

The majority of patients (n = 79, 68.1%) had uncomplicated appendicitis. Appendectomy was performed during the initial encounter in 64 (55.2%) patients and more extended bowel resection (including cecectomy, hemicolectomy, or stoma) in 8 (6.9%). Appendectomy was performed laparoscopically in 95% of cases.

The hospital day when the patient first underwent abdominal CT, MR, or US was used as the proxy for date of appendicitis diagnosis and was available in 107 patients (9 missing). First imaging occurred at a median of 2 days after admission (IQR 0–14). The median time from first imaging to surgery was 1 day (IQR 0–9.8), but in 26 patients surgery was delayed for more than 2 days after first imaging (20 appendectomy, 6 with bowel resection) (Fig. 16.1). In addition, 13 patients underwent delayed appendectomy during a subsequent encounter. In total 85 (73.3%) patients underwent surgery at some point during the study period, with 39 (33.6%) having early surgery, 39 (33.6%) having delayed surgery, and 7 (6.0%) having surgery during the initial admission with unknown timing.

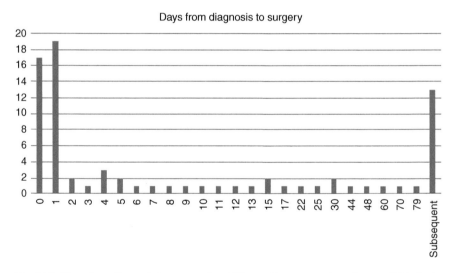

Days from diagnosis to surgery

Fig. 16.1 Days from diagnosis to surgery for children with neutropenia and appendicitis in the Pediatric Health Information System Database

For the eight patients who underwent bowel resection or enterostomy during the initial encounter, the majority ($n = 6$, 75%) had complicated appendicitis. Likewise, of 15 patients who underwent drain placement during the initial encounter, 10 (66%) had complicated appendicitis.

Discussion

Surgeons managing children with primary and secondary immune deficiencies who develop acute appendicitis must balance the risk of inadequate source control against the potential increased morbidity with surgical intervention. Although existing literature is limited, current evidence supports the safety and efficacy of early laparoscopic appendectomy, even in patients with a very low absolute neutrophil count. Historical concerns about infectious and surgical wound complications in children with neutropenia may be of less significance in the era of minimally invasive surgery, coupled with modern supportive care and antibiotic therapy. However, antibiotic therapy, either as a bridge to appendectomy after resolution of neutropenia or as a definitive treatment for appendicitis, seems to be a safe and effective alternative.

Findings from the Pediatric Health Information System Database mostly correlate with findings from institutional series. The rate of perforated appendicitis was 32% in the database study compared to 44% in the case series. Eighty percent of children in the PHIS study had a hematologic malignancy, echoing findings from the institutional series. The rate of early appendectomy was lower in the PHIS study compared to the case series, possibly because the PHIS data is more recent and reflects more current practice. The PHIS findings also correlate more closely with results from the multi-institutional series from France, which likewise had a lower rate of early appendectomy.

Current evidence is inadequate to recommend a definitive management algorithm. As always, the complete clinical picture must be taken into account. For this complex patient population, a multidisciplinary discussion between the surgical team and primary medical (e.g., hematology, transplant medicine, or infectious disease) team is advised. A key factor in the decision-making algorithm for children with appendicitis in the setting of a suppressed immune system is the expected duration of their immune suppression. When the immune deficiency is not anticipated to improve, as in children with primary immunodeficiency syndromes, then definitive treatment for appendicitis should be undertaken expeditiously. Conversely, in children expected to experience recovery of their immune system, delaying definitive management of their appendicitis may be considered. Patients who rapidly improve with antibiotic therapy may be considered for either definitive non-operative therapy or more commonly for delayed appendectomy following count recovery to avoid the risk of recurrence during subsequent episode of neutropenia. At the very least, treatment with antibiotics allows surgery to be delayed until modifiable issues are addressed. These might include treating concurrent thrombocytopenia, reducing levels of immunotherapy when clinically appropriate, or treating with a granulocyte colony-stimulating factor analog.

Further research is needed to truly understand the rates of wound and infectious complications in children with immune suppression in the era of minimally invasive surgery with modern antibiotics. In addition, current studies in immune competent patients assessing the success of non-operative appendicitis management will also help inform treatment decisions for these patients with immune deficiencies.

Conclusion

Even with an impaired ability to mount an immune response, often coupled with other complex comorbidities, most children with acute appendicitis do well. Timely diagnosis, multidisciplinary care, and treatment of modifiable comorbidities are key to avoiding excess morbidity.

Clinical Pearls

- Children with acute appendicitis in the setting of an immune deficiency, including neutropenia due to chemotherapy, can be safely managed with either immediate appendectomy or antibiotic therapy followed by appendectomy after count recovery.
- The role of definitive antibiotic treatment without surgery remains under investigation.

References

1. Hobson MJ, Carney DE, Molik KA, Vik T, Scherer LR 3rd, Rouse TM, et al. Appendicitis in childhood hematologic malignancies: analysis and comparison with typhlitis. J Pediatr Surg. 2005;40(1):214–9; discussion 9–20.
2. Scarpa AA, Hery G, Petit A, Brethon B, Jimenez I, Gandemer V, et al. Appendicitis in a neutropenic patient: a multicentric retrospective study. J Pediatr Hematol Oncol. 2017;39(5):365–9.
3. Chui CH, Chan MY, Tan AM, Low Y, Yap TL, Jacobsen AS. Appendicitis in immunosuppressed children: still a diagnostic and therapeutic dilemma? Pediatr Blood Cancer. 2008;50(6):1282–3.
4. Kim EY, Lee JW, Chung NG, Cho B, Kim HK, Chung JH. Acute appendicitis in children with acute leukemia: experiences of a single institution in Korea. Yonsei Med J. 2012;53(4):781–7.
5. Mortellaro VE, Juang D, Fike FB, Saites CG, Potter DD Jr, Iqbal CW, et al. Treatment of appendicitis in neutropenic children. J Surg Res. 2011;170(1):14–6.
6. Singer J, Stringel G, Ozkaynak MF, McBride W, Pandya S, Sandoval C. Laparoscopic surgery for acute appendicitis in children with cancer. JSLS. 2015;19(3):e2015.00066.
7. Warad D, Kohorst MA, Altaf S, Ishitani MB, Khan S, Rodriguez V, et al. Acute appendicitis in acute leukemia and the potential role of decitabine in the critically ill patient. Leuk Res Rep. 2015;4(1):21–3.
8. Wiegering VA, Kellenberger CJ, Bodmer N, Bergstraesser E, Niggli F, Grotzer M, et al. Conservative management of acute appendicitis in children with hematologic malignancies during chemotherapy-induced neutropenia. J Pediatr Hematol Oncol. 2008;30(6):464–7.
9. Shigemura T, Ohno Y, Sano K, Uehara T, Terada M, Koike K, et al. Gangrenous appendicitis in a patient with severe congenital neutropenia. Pediatr Int. 2016;58(10):1093–4.

Index

© Springer Nature Switzerland AG 2019
C. J. Hunter (ed.), *Controversies in Pediatric Appendicitis*,
https://doi.org/10.1007/978-3-030-15006-8

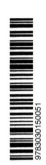

9783030150051